Workbook to Accompany

Cardiopulmonary
Anatomy and Physiology

Essentials for
Respiratory Care

Workbook to Accompany

Cardiopulmonary Anatomy and Physiology

Essentials for Respiratory Care

Third Edition

Terry Des Jardins, M.Ed., R.R.T.
Department of Respiratory Care
Parkland College
Champaign, Illinois

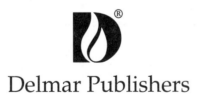

Delmar Publishers

an International Thomson Publishing company I(T)P®

Albany • Bonn • Boston • Cincinnati • Detroit • London • Madrid
Melbourne • Mexico City • New York • Pacific Grove • Paris • San Francisco
Singapore • Tokyo • Toronto • Washington

NOTICE TO THE READER

COPYRIGHT © 1998
by Delmar Publishers
a division of International Thomson Publishing Inc.

The ITP logo is a trademark under license.

Printed in the United States of America
For information, contact:

Delmar Publishers
3 Columbia Circle, Box 15015
Albany, NY 12212-5015

International Thomson Publishing Europe
Berkshire House
168-173 High Holborn
London, WC1V 7AA
England

Thomas Nelson Australia
102 Dodds Street
South Melbourne, 3205
Victoria, Australia

Nelson Canada
1120 Birchmount Road
Scarborough, Ontario
Canada, M1K 5G4

International Thomson Editores
Campos Eliseos 385, Piso 7
Col Polanco
11560 Mexico D F Mexico

International Thomson Publishing
GmbH
Konigswinterer Strasse 418
53227 Bonn
Germany

International Thomson Publishing Asia
221 Henderson Road
#05-10 Henderson Building
Singapore 0315

International Thomson Publishing—Japan
Hirakawacho Kyowa Building, 3F
2-2-1 Hirakawacho
Chiyoda-ku, Tokyo 102
Japan

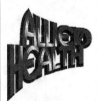
2 3 4 5 6 7 8 9 10 XXX 02 01 00 99 98

ISBN: 0-8273-8258-8
Library of Congress Catalog Card Number: 97-8797

CONTENTS

INTRODUCTION

This workbook is designed to enhance the learner's understanding, retention, and clinical application of the material presented in the textbook. The questions in the workbook parallel (in a step-by-step fashion) the information presented in the textbook. The student is asked to do such things as label and color illustrations, fill in the blanks, define terms, match answers, calculate equations, and write short answers. Answers to the questions, with page references to the textbook (a remedial-loop mechanism), appear at the end of the workbook.

The completed study questions serve as an excellent study tool to help the student review and prepare for chapter quizzes and exams. This workbook also gives the reader an opportunity to evaluate the degree of mastery of the material presented in the text. Although answering 75 percent of the questions correctly is considered an acceptable mastery level, study and review should continue until greater than 90 percent accuracy has been achieved. The student may wish to copy and maintain unanswered questions of various sections of the workbook for reuse and periodic self-assessment.

Terry Des Jardins

CHAPTER ONE

THE ANATOMY OF THE RESPIRATORY SYSTEM

THE UPPER AIRWAY

1. Label and color the following structures of the upper airway:

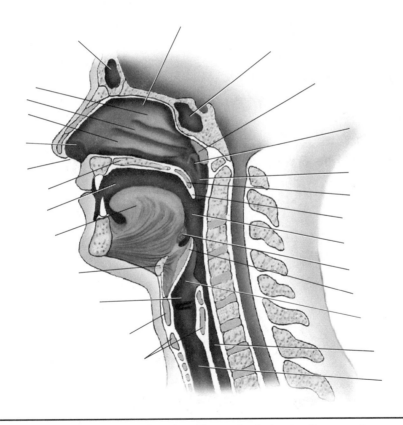

Figure 1–1 *Sagittal section of human head, showing the upper airway.*

2. The primary function(s) of the upper airway are:

    a. _____

    _____

    b. _____

    _____

    c. _____

    _____

3. The primary functions of the nose are to do the following to inspired air:

    a. _____

    _____

    b. _____

    _____

    c. _____

    _____

4. Label and color the following structures that form the outer portion of the nose:

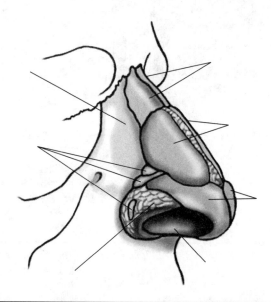

Figure 1–2   *Structure of the nose.*

5. Label and color the following structures of the internal portion of the nose:

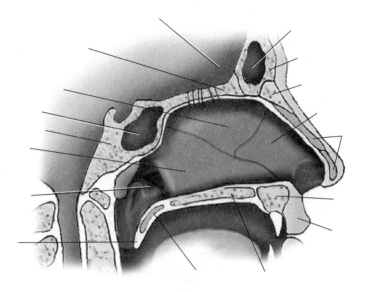

Figure 1–3   *Sagittal section through the nose, showing the parts of the nasal septum.*

6. _____ epithelium lines the posterior two-thirds of the nasal cavity.

7. List the three bony protrusions in the nasal cavity that increase the contact time between the inspired air and the warm, moist surface of the nasal cavity:

   a. _____

   _____

   b. _____

   _____

   c. _____

   _____

8. Label and color the following sinuses of the skull:

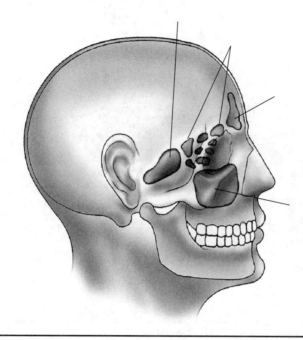

Figure 1–4 *Lateral view of head, showing sinuses.*

9. The _____ muscle elevates the soft palate.

10. The **oral cavity** is lined with _____ epithelium.

11. The **palatine arches** are composed of the _____ arch

    and the _____ arch.

12. The **nasopharynx** is lined with _____
    epithelium.

13. The _____ serves to equalize the pressure between
    the nasopharynx and the middle ear.

14. The **oropharynx** is lined with _____ epithelium.

15. The **laryngopharynx** is lined with _____ epithelium.

16. Label and color the following structures of the oral cavity:

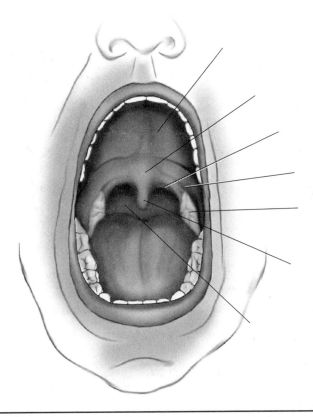

Figure 1–5 *Oral cavity.*

THE LOWER AIRWAYS

1. Functionally, the **larynx**:

    a. _____

    _____

    b. _____

    _____

    c. _____

    _____

2. Label and color the following cartilages of the larynx:

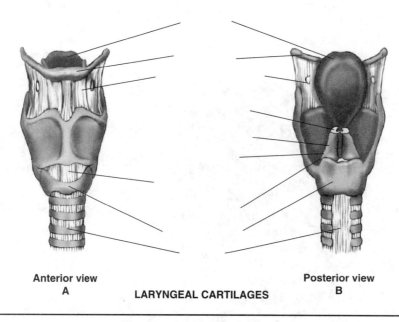

Anterior view
A
LARYNGEAL CARTILAGES
Posterior view
B

Figure 1–6   *Cartilages of the larynx.*

3. Label and color the structures observed in the superior view of the vocal folds:

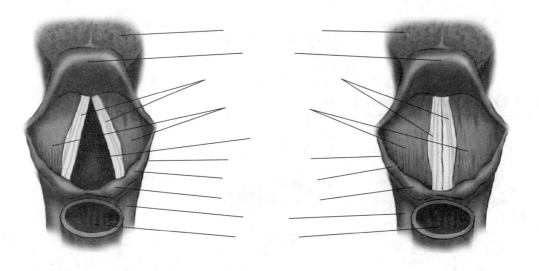

Figure 1–7   *Superior view of vocal folds (cords).*

4. The elastic tissue that forms the medial border of each vocal fold is called the _____

_____ .

5. Anteriorly, the vocal cords attach to the posterior surface of the _____

_____ .

6. The space between the vocal cords is called the _____

or the _____ .

7. Above the vocal cords, the laryngeal mucosa is composed of _____

_____ epithelium.

8. Below the vocal cords, the laryngeal mucosa is lined with _____

_____ epithelium.

9. An expiratory effort against a closed glottis (e.g., during physical work such as lifting or pushing)

is known as _____ .

10. Label and color the following **extrinsic laryngeal** muscles:

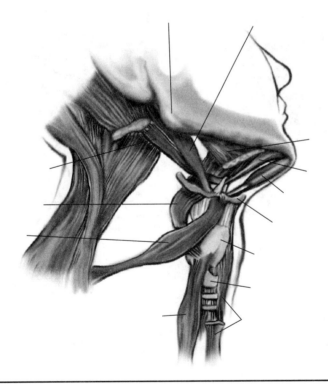

Figure 1–8 *Extrinsic laryngeal muscles.*

11. Label and color the following **intrinsic muscles** of the larynx:

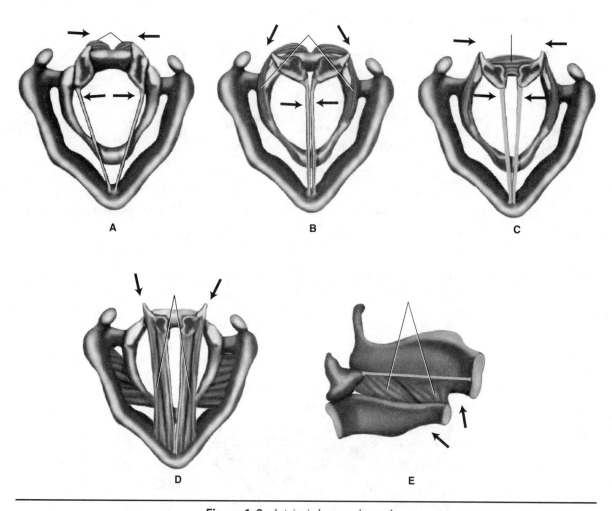

Figure 1–9 *Intrinsic laryngeal muscles.*

THE TRACHEOBRONCHIAL TREE

1. Label and color the following structures of the tracheobronchial tree:

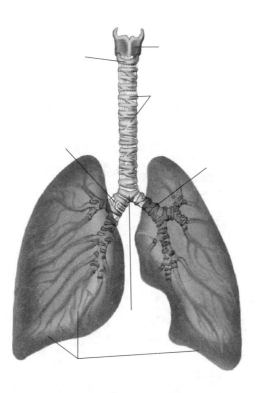

Figure 1–10 *Tracheobronchial tree.*

2. The tracheobronchial tree is composed of the following three layers:

   a. _____

   _____

   b. _____

   _____

   c. _____

   _____

3. The epithelial lining of the tracheobronchial tree is mainly composed of _____

   _____ epithelium.

4. Most of the mucus that lines the lumen of the tracheobronchial tree is produced by the

   _____ .

5. The two distinct layers of the mucous blanket are the _____

   and the _____ .

6. Label and color the following section of epithelial lining of the tracheobronchial tree:

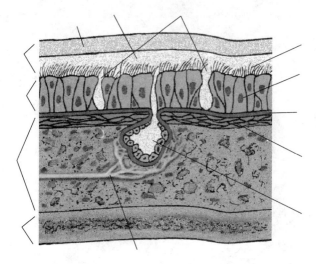

Figure 1–11   *Epithelial lining of the tracheobronchial tree.*

7. List factors that are known to slow the rate of the mucociliary transport mechanism:

   a. _____

   b. _____

   c. _____

   d. _____

   e. _____

   f. _____

   g. _____

   h. _____

   i. _____

8. List five chemical mediators of inflammation secreted by the mast cell:

   a. _____

   b. _____

   c. _____

   d. _____

   e. _____

9. The adult trachea is about _____ to _____ cm long and _____ to _____ cm in diameter.

10. The bifurcation of the trachea is known as the _____ .

11. In the adult, the right main stem bronchus branches off the vertical trachea at about a _____
    -degree angle; the left main stem bronchus forms a _____ to _____ -degree angle with the vertical
    trachea.

12. **Canals of Lambert** are found in the _____ of the
    tracheobronchial tree.

13. From the trachea to the terminal bronchioles, the total cross-sectional area of the tracheobronchial
    tree progressively _____ .

14. The bronchial arteries nourish the tracheobronchial tree down to, and including, the _____
    _____ .

15. In addition to the tracheobronchial tree, the bronchial arteries nourish the

    _____

    _____

    _____

    _____

16. Approximately one-third of the bronchial venous blood returns to the right atrium by way of the

    _____

    _____

17. About two-thirds of the bronchial venous blood empties into the pulmonary circulation by means

    of _____

    _____

THE SITES OF GAS EXCHANGE

1. The anatomic structures distal to the terminal bronchioles consist of the

   a. _____ bronchioles

   b. _____ ducts

   c. _____ sacs

2. Using the following schematic drawing, label the following anatomic structures distal to the terminal bronchiole:

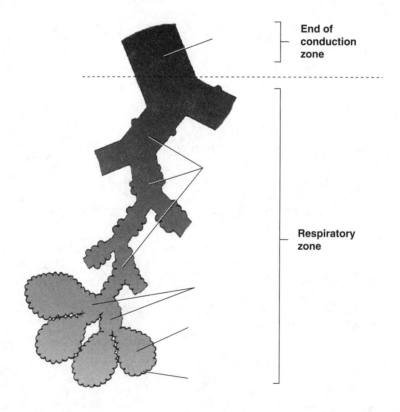

Figure 1–12   *Schematic drawing of the anatomic structures distal to the terminal bronchioles; collectively, these are referred to as the primary lobule.*

3. Label and color the following components of the alveolar-capillary network:

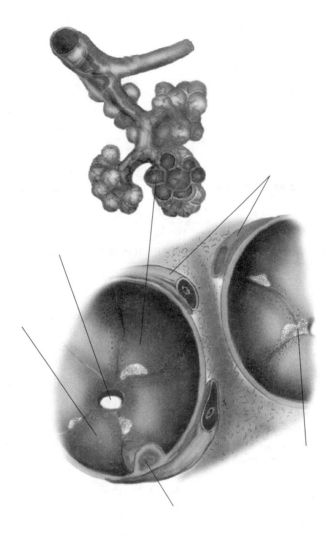

Figure 1–13 *Alveolar-capillary network.*

4. In the adult lung, there are approximately _____ million alveoli.

5. The average surface area of the adult lung is _____ square meters.

6. A **primary lobule** consists of which structures distal to a single terminal bronchiole?

_____

_____

7. There are approximately _____ primary lobules in the lung.

8. Synonyms of a primary lobule are

    a. _____

    b. _____

    c. _____

    d. _____

9. The **Type I cell** found in the alveolar epithelium is also called a _____

    _____ .

10. The **Type II cell** found in the alveolar epithelium is also called a _____

    _____ .

11. The Type I cells form about _____ percent of the alveolar substance.

12. The _____ cells are believed to be the primary source of pulmonary surfactant.

13. Small holes in the walls of the interalveolar septa are called _____

    _____ .

14. The _____ play a major role in removing foreign
    particles that are deposited within the acini.

15. The two major compartments of the interstitium are the _____

    and the _____ .

PULMONARY VASCULAR SYSTEM AND LYMPHATIC SYSTEM

1. Using the following schematic drawing, label and color the components of the major blood vessels:

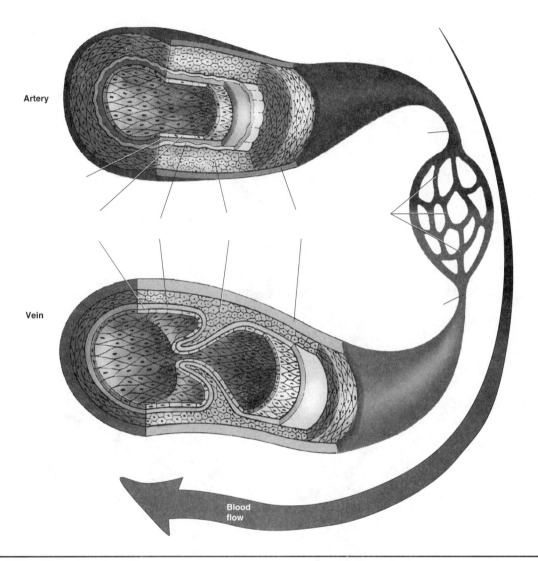

Artery

Vein

Blood flow

Figure 1–14 *Schematic drawing of the components of the major blood vessels.*

2. The arterioles play an important role in the distribution and regulation of blood and are called

   the _____ vessels.

3. The walls of the pulmonary capillaries are less than _____ thick and the external

   diameter is about _____ .

4. Because the veins are capable of collecting a large amount of blood with very little pressure change, the veins are called _____ vessels.

5. Superficially, lymphatic vessels are found around the lung just beneath the _____

_____ .

6. Within the lungs, the lymphatic vessels arise from the _____

_____ .

7. Label the following lymph nodes associated with the trachea and the right and left main stem bronchi:

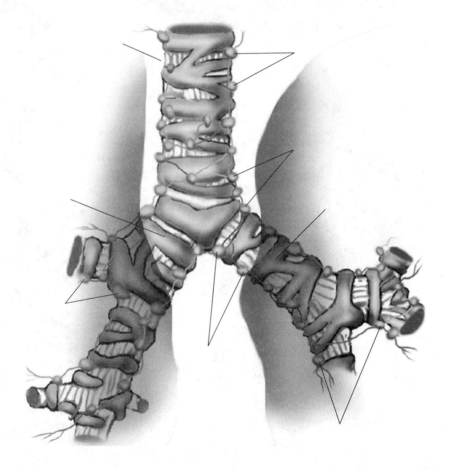

Figure 1–15   *Lymph nodes associated with the trachea and the right and left main stem bronchi.*

NEURAL CONTROL OF THE LUNGS

1. The smooth muscle that surrounds the bronchi and arterioles is controlled by the _____

   _____ .

2. Compare and contrast the effects of the sympathetic and parasympathetic nervous system on the following effector sites:

TABLE 1–1   Some Effects of Autonomic Nervous System Activity

EFFECTOR SITE	SYMPATHETIC NERVOUS SYSTEM	PARASYMPATHETIC NERVOUS SYSTEM
Heart		
Bronchial smooth muscle		
Bronchial glands		
Salivary glands		
Stomach		
Intestines		
Eye		

3. When the sympathetic nervous system is activated, _____

   or _____ neural transmitters are released.

4. When the **beta$_2$ receptors** are stimulated, the bronchial smooth muscles _____

   _____ .

5. When the **alpha receptors** are stimulated, the smooth muscles of the arterioles _____

   _____ .

6. When the parasympathetic nervous system is activated, the neural transmitter _____

   _____ is released.

THE LUNGS

1. The apex of the lungs rise to about the level of the _____ rib.

2. Anteriorly, the base of the lungs external to about the level of the _____ rib, and posteriorly to about the level of the _____ rib.

3. At the center of the mediastinal border, the right and left main stem bronchi, blood vessels, lymph vessels, and various nerves enter and exit the lungs through the _____ .

4. In the right lung, the **oblique fissure** extends from the _____ to the _____ borders.

5. In the right lung, the **horizontal fissure** extends horizontally from the _____ to about the level of the _____ costal cartilage.

6. In the left lung, the **oblique fissure** extends from the _____ to the _____ borders of the lung.

7. Label the following structures of the anterior portion of the lungs:

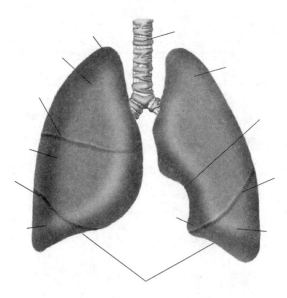

Figure 1–16 *Anterior view of the lungs.*

8. Label the following structures of the medial portion of the lungs:

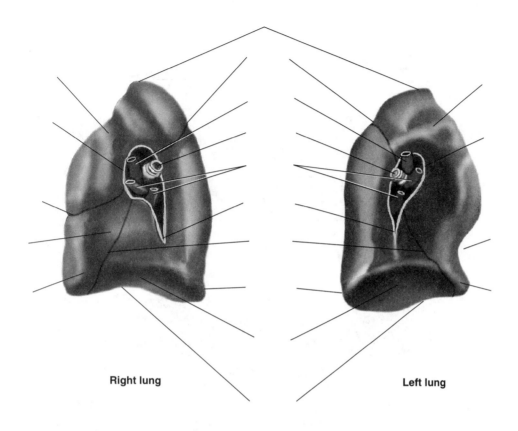

Right lung   **Left lung**

Figure 1–17 *Medial view of the lungs.*

9. Match the number of the lung segments shown in the box to the different views of the lung. Content retention is also enhanced when the lung segments are colored.

Right lung		Left lung	
Upper lobe		**Upper lobe**	
Apical	1	Upper division	
Posterior	2	Apical/Posterior	1 & 2
Anterior	3	Anterior	3
Middle lobe		**Lower division (lingular)**	
Lateral	4	Superior lingula	4
Medial	5	Inferior lingula	5
Lower lobe		**Lower lobe**	
Superior	6	Superior	6
Medial basal	7	Anterior medial	7 & 8
Anterior basal	8	Lateral basal	9
Lateral basal	9	Posterior basal	10
Posterior basal	10		

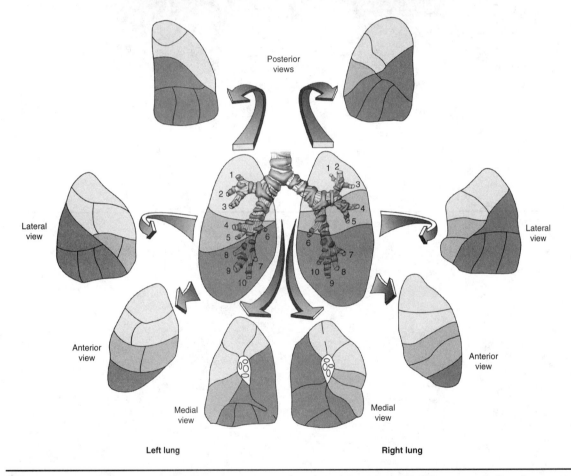

Figure 1–18 *Lung segments. Although the segment subdivisions of the right and left lungs are similar, there are some slight anatomic differences, which are noted by combined names and numbers. Because of these slight variations, some workers consider that, technically, there are only eight segments in the left lung and that the apical-posterior segment is number 1 and the anteromedial is number 6.*

10. Label the following major structures around the lungs:

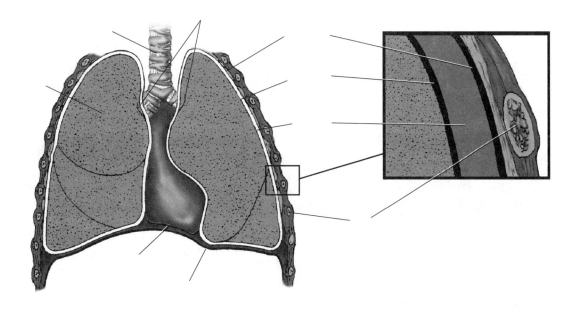

Figure 1–19 *Major structures around the lungs.*

THE MEDIASTINUM, PLEURAL MEMBRANES, AND THORAX

1. List the anatomic structures that are contained in, or pass through, the **mediastinum**:

   _____

   _____

   _____

2. The _____ pleura is firmly attached to the outer surface of each lung.

3. The _____ pleura lines the inside of the thoracic walls.

4. The potential space between the pleural membranes is called the _____

   _____ .

5. List the three major structures that compose the sternum:

   a. _____

   b. _____

   c. _____

6. The first seven ribs are called the _____ .

7. Ribs eight, nine and ten are referred to as the _____ ribs.

8. Ribs eleven and twelve are called the _____ ribs.

9. Label the following components of the thorax:

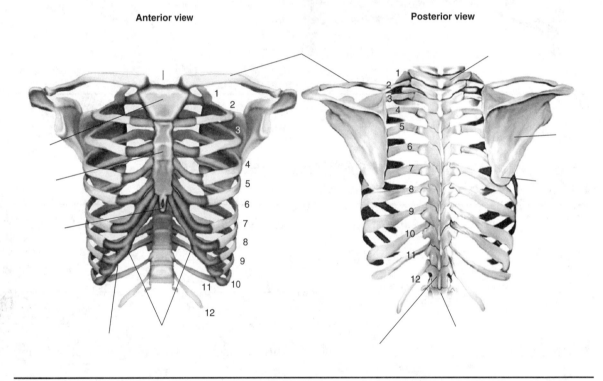

Figure 1–20 *The thorax.*

10. Label the following components of the intercostal space:

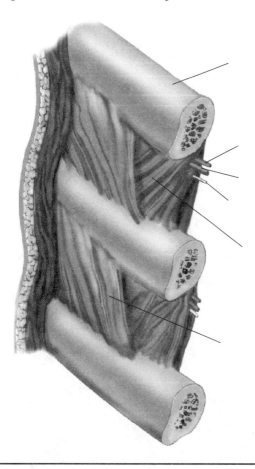

Figure 1–21   *The intercostal space.*

THE DIAPHRAGM

1. Each hemidiaphragm merges together at the midline into a broad connective sheet called the

   _____ .

2. List the structures that pierce the diaphragm:

   _____

   _____

3. The _____ nerves supply the primary motor innervation to each hemidiaphragm.

4. When used as accessory muscles for inspiration, the **scalene muscles** elevate the

_____ and _____ ribs.

5. When used as accessory muscles of inspiration, the **sternocleidomastoid muscles** elevate the

_____ .

6. When used as accessory muscles of inspiration, the **pectoralis major muscles** elevate the

_____ , causing an increased _____

diameter.

7. Normally, the **trapezius** rotates the _____ , raises the _____ ,

and abducts and flexes the _____ .

8. During inspiration, the **external intercostal muscles** pull the ribs _____ and

_____ .

9. Label and color the following accessory muscles of expiration:

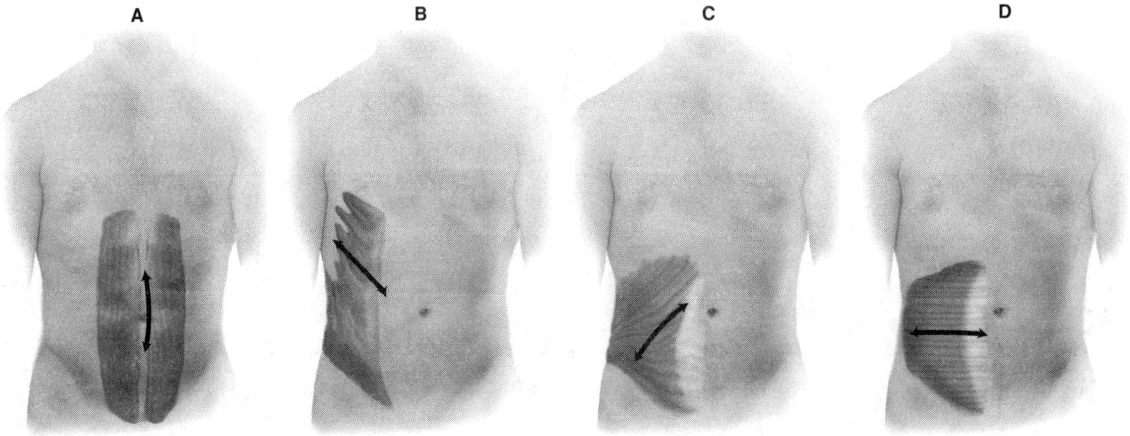

Figure 1–22   *Accessory muscles of expiration.*

10. During exhalation, the **internal intercostal muscles** pull the ribs _____ and

_____ .

CHAPTER TWO

VENTILATION

PRESSURE DIFFERENCES ACROSS THE LUNGS

1. The pressure difference between two points in a tube or vessel is called the _____ .

2. The barometric pressure difference between the mouth pressure and alveolar pressure is called the _____ .

3. The difference between the alveolar pressure and the pleural pressure is called the _____ .

4. The difference between the alveolar pressure and the body surface pressure is called the _____ .

5. If the gas pressure at the beginning of a vessel is 12 mm Hg and the pressure at the other end of the same vessel is 7 mm Hg, what is the driving pressure?

Answer: _____

6. If the P_{alv} is 751 mm Hg and the P_m is 758 mm Hg, what is the P_{ta}?

Answer: _____

7. If the P_{pl} is 752 mm Hg and the P_{alv} is 748 mm Hg, what is the P_{tp}?

Answer: _____

8. If the P_{alv} is 751 mm Hg and the P_{bs} is 757 mm Hg, what is the P_{tt}?

Answer: _____

9. During inspiration, the thoracic volume increases and the intrapleural and intra-alveolar pressures

_____ .

10. During expiration, the intra-alveolar pressure is (_____ greater; _____ lower) than the barometric pressure.

11. During a normal expiration, the intrapleural pressure is always (_____ above; _____ below) the barometric pressure.

12. The normal intrapleural pressure change is about _____ to _____ cm H_2O pressure, or _____ to _____ mm Hg.

STATIC CHARACTERISTICS OF THE LUNGS

1. The term **static** refers to _____

   _____

   _____

2. The lungs have a natural tendency to (_____ collapse; _____ expand).

3. The chest wall has a natural tendency to (_____ collapse; _____ expand).

4. The two major static forces of the lungs are:

   a. _____

   b. _____

ELASTIC PROPERTIES OF THE LUNGS

1. **Lung compliance** is defined as the change in lung _____ per change in _____

   _____ .

2. **Case A**

   a. If an individual generates an intrapleural pressure of -7 cm H_2O during inspiration, and the lungs accept a new volume of 385 ml of air, what is the compliance of the lungs?

   Answer: _____

b. If the same patient, four hours later, generates an intrapleural pressure of -5 cm H_2O during inspiration, and the lungs accept a new volume of 350 ml of air, what is the compliance of the lungs?

Answer: _____

c. The lung compliance of the above patient is (check one): increasing _____ decreasing _____

3. **Case B**

a. If a mechanical ventilator generates a $+9$ cm H_2O pressure during inspiration and the lungs accept a new volume of 450 ml of gas, what is the compliance of the lungs?

Answer: _____

b. If, on the same patient six hours later, the mechanical ventilator generates a $+15$ cm H_2O pressure and the lungs accept a new volume of 675 ml of gas, what is the compliance of the lungs?

Answer: _____

c. Compare the answers to the first two questions (a & b) above. The patient's lung compliance is

(check one): increasing _____ decreasing _____

4. Under normal resting conditions, the average lung compliance during each breath is approximately

_____ .

5. According to the following volume-pressure curve, if an individual has a resting lung volume of 1500 ml, and generates a negative 25 cm H_2O pressure (in addition to the negative pressure required to maintain the resting lung volume), how many ml of gas will the lungs accommodate (in addition to the resting lung volume)?

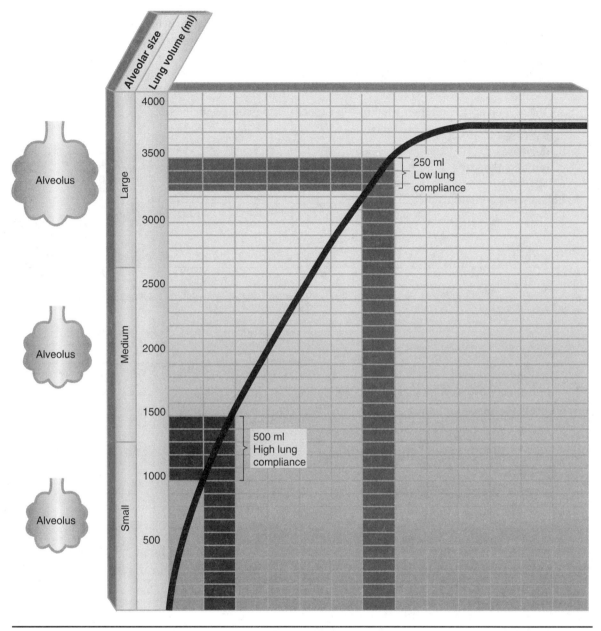

Figure 2–1 *Normal volume-pressure curve. The curve shows that lung compliance progressively decreases as the lungs expand in response to more volume. For example, note the greater volume change between 5 and 10 cm H_2O (small/ medium alveoli) than between 30 and 35 cm H_2O (large alveoli).*

Answer: _____

6. When lung compliance decreases, the volume-pressure curve moves to the _____ .

7. When the volume-pressure curve moves to the left, lung compliance is (circle one):

   a. increased
   b. decreased
   c. unchanged

8. As the alveoli approach their total filling capacity, lung compliance:

   a. increases
   b. decreases
   c. remains the same

9. **Elastance** is defined as the _____

   _____

   _____

   _____

   _____

   _____

10. In pulmonary physiology, elastance is defined as _____
    and is expressed as:

    Elastance =

11. Lungs with high compliance have _____ elastance, and lungs with low compliance

    have _____ elastance.

12. **Hooke's law** states that _____

_____

_____

_____

_____

_____

13. When Hooke's law is applied to the elastic properties of the lungs, _____ is

substituted for length and _____ is substituted for force.

14. The molecular, cohesive force at the liquid–gas interface is called _____ .

15. The liquid film that lines the interior surface of the alveoli has the potential to exert a force of

_____ .

16. When Laplace's law is applied to a sphere with one liquid–gas interface, the equation is written as follows:

    P =

17. The mathematical arrangement of Laplace's law shows that the distending pressure of a liquid bubble is

    a. _____

    _____

    and

    b. _____

    _____

18. According to Laplace's law, as the surface tension of a liquid bubble increases, the distending pressure required to hold the bubble open _____ ; and as the radius of the bubble increases, the distending pressure _____ .

19. When two different size bubbles with the same surface tension are in direct communication the:
    a. larger bubble will empty into the smaller bubble
    b. smaller bubble will empty into the larger bubble
    c. distending pressures in the two bubbles are equal; thus, there is no gas flow between the two bubbles.

20. During the formation of a new bubble, the principles of Laplace's law do not come into effect until the distending pressure of the liquid sphere goes beyond the _____ .

21. As a liquid bubble increases in size, the surface tension:
    a. increases
    b. decreases
    c. remains the same

22. **Pulmonary surfactant** is produced by the _____ .

23. The surfactant molecule has both a hydrophobic end, which means it is _____ , and a hydrophilic end, which means it is _____ .

24. In the healthy lung, when the alveolus decreases in size, the amount of surfactant to alveolar surface area _____ . This action causes the alveolar surface tension to _____ .

25. It is estimated that the surface tension of the average alveolus varies from _____ in the small alveolus to about _____ in the fully distended alveolus.

26. List some general causes of surfactant deficiency:

    a. _____

    b. _____

    c. _____

    d. _____

    e. _____

27. In the healthy lung, both the elastic force and the surface tension force are (_____ low; _____ high) in the small alveolus.

DYNAMIC CHARACTERISTICS OF THE LUNGS

1. The term **dynamic** is defined as the _____

   _____

2. In the lungs, dynamic refers to _____

   _____

3. When **Poiseuille's law** is arranged for flow $\dot{V}$, it is written as follows:

   $\dot{V} =$

4. According to Poiseuille's law, and assuming all other variables remain the same:

   a. as the pressure increases, flow (_____ increases; _____ decreases)

   b. as the length of a tube decreases, flow (_____ increases; _____ decreases)

   c. as the radius of a tube increases, flow (_____ increases; _____ decreases)

   d. as the viscosity decreases, flow (_____ increases; _____ decreases)

5. Using Poiseuille's law equations and assuming all other variables remain the same, answer the following questions:

   a. If the radius of a tube, that has gas flowing through it at 32 liters per minute (L/min) is reduced by 50 percent of its original size, what will be the new gas flow through the tube?

   Answer: _____

b. If the radius of a tube that has gas flowing through it at 28 L/min is reduced by 16 percent, what will be the new gas flow through the tube?

Answer: _____

c. If the radius of a tube that has a driving pressure of 16 cm H_2O is reduced by 50 percent of its original size, what will be the new driving pressure required to maintain the same gas flow through the tube?

Answer: _____

d. If the radius of a tube that has a driving pressure of 10 cm H_2O is reduced by 16 percent of its original size, what will be the new driving pressure required to maintain the same gas flow through the tube?

Answer: _____

e. If the radius of a tube that has gas flowing through it at 50 L/min is increased by 50 percent of its original size, what will be the new gas flow through the tube?

Answer: _____

27. In the healthy lung, both the elastic force and the surface tension force are (_____ low; _____ high) in the small alveolus.

DYNAMIC CHARACTERISTICS OF THE LUNGS

1. The term **dynamic** is defined as the _____

   _____

2. In the lungs, dynamic refers to _____

   _____

3. When **Poiseuille's law** is arranged for flow $\dot{V}$, it is written as follows:

   $\dot{V} =$

4. According to Poiseuille's law, and assuming all other variables remain the same:

   a. as the pressure increases, flow (_____ increases; _____ decreases)

   b. as the length of a tube decreases, flow (_____ increases; _____ decreases)

   c. as the radius of a tube increases, flow (_____ increases; _____ decreases)

   d. as the viscosity decreases, flow (_____ increases; _____ decreases)

5. Using Poiseuille's law equations and assuming all other variables remain the same, answer the following questions:

   a. If the radius of a tube, that has gas flowing through it at 32 liters per minute (L/min) is reduced by 50 percent of its original size, what will be the new gas flow through the tube?

   Answer: _____

b. If the radius of a tube that has gas flowing through it at 28 L/min is reduced by 16 percent, what will be the new gas flow through the tube?

Answer: _____

c. If the radius of a tube that has a driving pressure of 16 cm H_2O is reduced by 50 percent of its original size, what will be the new driving pressure required to maintain the same gas flow through the tube?

Answer: _____

d. If the radius of a tube that has a driving pressure of 10 cm H_2O is reduced by 16 percent of its original size, what will be the new driving pressure required to maintain the same gas flow through the tube?

Answer: _____

e. If the radius of a tube that has gas flowing through it at 50 L/min is increased by 50 percent of its original size, what will be the new gas flow through the tube?

Answer: _____

f. If the radius of a tube that has gas flowing through it at 100 L/min is increased by 16 percent of its original size, what will be the new gas flow through the tube?

Answer: _____

g. If the radius of a tube that has a driving pressure of 80 cm H_2O is increased by 50 percent of its original size, what will be the new driving pressure required to maintain the same gas flow through the tube?

Answer: _____

h. If the radius of a tube that has a driving pressure of 5 cm H_2O, is increased by 16 percent of its original size, what will be the new driving pressure required to maintain the same gas flow through the tube?

Answer: _____

6. Write the simple proportionalities of Poiseuille's law for flow ($\dot{V}$) and pressure (P):

$\dot{V}$=

P =

AIRWAY RESISTANCE AND DYNAMIC COMPLIANCE

1. Airway resistance (R_{aw}) is defined as the _____

_____

_____

2. Write the equation for airway resistance (R_{aw}) and include the units of measurement:

R_{aw} =

3. If a patient produces a flow rate of 10 liters per second (L/sec) during inspiration by generating a transairway pressure (P_{ta}) of 30 cm H_2O, what is the patient's R_{aw}?

Answer: _____

4. The normal R_{aw} in the tracheobronchial tree is about _____ to _____ cm $H_2O/L/sec$.

5. **Laminar** gas flow refers to _____

_____

6. **Turbulent** gas flow refers to _____

_____

7. **Time constant** is defined as the _____

_____

_____

8. Lung regions that have an increased airway resistance, require:

   a. less time to inflate
   b. more time to inflate
   c. no change in time to inflate

9. Lung regions that have an increased compliance, require:

    a. less time to inflate
    b. more time to inflate
    c. no change in time to inflate

10. Which of the following cause lung regions to have a long time constant?

    I. Decreased airway resistance
    II. Increased lung compliance
    III. Increased airway resistance
    IV. Decreased lung compliance

        a. I only
        b. III only
        c. II and III only
        d. III and IV only
        e. II, III, and IV only

11. Lung regions that have a decreased airway resistance, require:

    a. less time to inflate
    b. more time to inflate
    c. no change in time to inflate

12. Lung regions that have a decreased compliance, require:

    a. less time to inflate
    b. more time to inflate
    c. no change in time to inflate

13. Which of the following cause lung regions to have a short time constant?

    I. Increased airway resistance
    II. Decreased lung compliance
    III. Decreased airway resistance
    IV. Increased lung compliance

        a. II only
        b. IV only
        c. III only
        d. I and IV only
        e. II and III only

14. **Dynamic compliance** is defined as the _____

_____

_____

_____

15. In the normal lung, the dynamic compliance is (_____ equal to; _____ greater than; _____ less than) static compliance at all breathing frequencies.

16. In the partially obstructed airways, the ratio of dynamic compliance to static compliance (_____ increases; _____ decreases; _____ remains the same) as the breathing frequency increases.

17. **Frequency dependent** refers to _____

_____

_____

_____

_____

VENTILATORY PATTERNS

1. The **ventilatory pattern** consists of the following three components:

   a. _____

   b. _____

   c. _____

2. The normal tidal volume is about _____ to _____ ml/kg; or _____ to _____ ml/lb.

3. The normal adult ventilatory rate is about _____ breaths per minute.

4. The normal I : E is about _____ : _____.

5. The gas that reaches the alveoli during inspiration is referred to as _____.

6. The gas that does not reach the alveoli during inspiration is referred to as _____

   _____.

7. **Anatomic dead space** is defined as _____

_____

_____

_____

8. If a patient weighs 130 pounds, about how many milliliters (ml) of inspired gas during each breath would be anatomic deadspace gas?

   Answer: _____

9. **Alveolar ventilation** is equal to the _____ minus the _____

   multiplied by the _____ .

10. If an individual presents with this data:

    - $V_T = 575$ ml
    - $V_D = 185$ ml
    - Breaths/minute = 16

    What is the alveolar ventilation?

    Answer: _____

11. **Alveolar dead space** is defined as _____

    _____

    _____

12. **Physiologic dead space** is defined as _____

    _____

13. In the upright position, the negative intrapleural pressure at the apex of the lung is normally (_____

    less; _____ greater) than at the base.

14. In the upright position, the alveoli in the upper lung regions are (_____ smaller; _____ larger;

    _____ equal) in size compared to the alveoli in the lower lung regions.

15. In the upright lung, ventilation is much greater in the:

    a. upper lung regions
    b. middle lung regions
    c. lower lung regions

16. When lung compliance decreases, the patient's ventilatory rate generally (_____ increases; _____ decreases; _____ remains the same) and the tidal volume (_____ increases; _____ decreases; _____ remains the same).

17. When airway resistance increases, the patient's ventilatory rate generally (_____ increases; _____ decreases; _____ remains the same) and the tidal volume (_____ increases; _____ decreases; _____ remains the same).

18. In response to a certain respiratory disorder, the patient may adopt a ventilatory pattern based on the expenditure of _____ rather than the efficiency of _____ .

19. **Apnea** is defined as the _____

    _____

20. **Eupnea** is defined as _____

    _____

21. **Biot's breathing** is defined as _____

    _____

    _____

    _____

22. **Hyperpnea** is defined as _____

    _____

    _____

23. **Hyperventilation** is defined as _____

_____

_____

_____

24. **Hypoventilation** is defined as _____

_____

_____

_____

25. **Tachypnea** is defined as _____

_____

26. **Cheyne-Stokes breathing** is defined as _____

_____

_____

_____

_____

27. **Kussmaul breathing** is defined as _____

_____

_____

28. **Orthopnea** is defined as _____

_____

_____

_____

29. **Dyspnea** is defined as _____

_____

_____

CHAPTER THREE

THE DIFFUSION
OF PULMONARY GASES

DIFFUSION AND GAS LAWS

1. **Diffusion** is defined as _____

_____

_____

2. **Boyle's law** states that _____

_____

_____

3. Boyle's law is written as follows:

4. If an airtight container, which has a volume of 400 ml and a pressure of 50 cm H_2O, has its volume reduced to 300 ml, what will be the new pressure in the container?

Answer: _____

5. If an airtight container, which has a volume of 55 ml and a pressure of 75 cm H_2O, has its volume increased to 110 ml, what will be the new pressure in the container?

Answer: _____

6. **Charles' law** states that _____

_____

_____

_____

7. Charles' law is written as follows:

8. If the temperature of gas in an 8-liter balloon is increased from 290 Kelvin to 340 Kelvin, what will be the new volume in the balloon?

Answer: _____

9. If the temperature of an automobile tire, which has 4.5 liters of air in it, is increased from 32° Celsius to 42° Celsius, what will be the new volume of gas (air) in the tire?

Answer: _____

10. **Gay-Lussac's law** states that _____

_____

_____

_____

11. Gay-Lussac's law is written as follows:

12. If the temperature of gas in a closed container, which has a pressure of 15 cm H_2O, is increased from 360 Kelvin to 375 Kelvin, what will be the new pressure in the container?

Answer: _____

13. If the temperature of the gas in a closed container, which has a pressure of 46 cm H_2O, is decreased from 40° Celsius to 30° Celsius, what will be the new pressure in the container?

Answer: _____

14. **Dalton's law** states that _____

_____

_____

_____

15. The following gases and their respective pressures are enclosed in a container:

GAS	PARTIAL PRESSURE
Nitrogen	470 mm Hg
Oxygen	130 mm Hg
Carbon Dioxide	50 mm Hg

According to Dalton's law, what is the total pressure in the container?

Answer: _____

THE PARTIAL PRESSURES OF ATMOSPHERIC GASES

1. At sea level, identify the percentage of the atmosphere and the partial pressure of the following gases that compose the barometric pressure:

TABLE 3–1   **Gases that Compose the Barometric Pressure**

GAS	% OF ATMOSPHERE	PARTIAL PRESSURE (mm Hg)
Nitrogen (N_2)		
Oxygen (O_2)		
Argon (Ar)		
Carbon Dioxide (CO_2)		

2. As one ascends a mountain, the barometric pressure (_____ increases; _____ decreases; _____ remains the same) and the percent concentration of oxygen (_____ increases; _____ decreases; _____ remains the same).

3. Compare and contrast the partial pressure of gases in the dry air, alveoli, arterial blood, and venous blood:

TABLE 3–2   **Partial Pressure (in mm Hg) of Gases in the Air, Alveoli, and Blood**

GASES	DRY AIR	ALVEOLAR GAS	ARTERIAL BLOOD	VENOUS BLOOD
P_{O_2}				
P_{CO_2}				
P_{H_2O} (water vapor)				
P_{N_2} (and other gases in minute quantities)				
Total				

4. The reason the partial pressure of oxygen in the atmosphere is so much higher than the partial pressure of oxygen in the alveoli is because

_____

_____

_____

_____

5. At body temperature, the alveolar gas has an absolute humidity of _____ and a water

 vapor pressure (P_{H_2O}) of _____ .

6. If a patient is receiving an $F_{I_{O_2}}$ of .70 on a day when the barometric pressure is 748 mm Hg, and if the Pa_{CO_2} is 50 mm Hg, what is the patient's alveolar oxygen tension ($P_{A_{O_2}}$)?

 Answer: _____

THE DIFFUSION OF PULMONARY GASES

1. List the structures of the alveolar-capillary membrane that gas molecules must diffuse through:

 a. _____

 b. _____

 c. _____

 d. _____

 e. _____

 f. _____

 g. _____

 h. _____

 i. _____

2. The thickness of the alveolar-capillary membrane is between _____ to

   _____ .

3. In the healthy resting person, the average $P\bar{v}_{O_2}$ is _____ mm Hg and the average $P\bar{v}_{CO_2}$ is

   _____ mm Hg.

4. Under normal circumstances, when venous blood enters the alveolar-capillary system, there is an

   oxygen pressure gradient of about _____ mm Hg, and a carbon dioxide pressure gradient of

   about _____ mm Hg.

5. The equilibrium of oxygen and carbon dioxide in the alveolar-capillary system is usually accom-

   plished in about _____ seconds.

6. The total transit time for blood to move through the alveolar-capillary system is about

   _____ seconds, which is about _____ of the time available.

7. During exercise, the time available for gas diffusion (circle one):

   a. increases
   b. decreases
   c. remains the same

8. **Fick's law** is written as follows:

   $\dot{V}$ gas =

9. According to Fick's law, as the

   a. thickness decreases, gas diffusion (circle one):

      a. increases
      b. decreases
      c. remains the same

   b. pressure difference increases, gas diffusion:

      a. increases
      b. decreases
      c. remains the same

   c. area decreases, gas diffusion:

     a. increases

     b. decreases

     c. remains the same

10. **Henry's law** states that: _____

_____

_____

_____

11. The amount of gas that can be dissolved by 1 ml of a given liquid at standard pressure and speci-

    fied temperature is known as the _____ .

12. **Graham's law** states that the rate of diffusion of a gas through a liquid is

   a. _____

_____

_____

   and

   b. _____

_____

PERFUSION- AND DIFFUSION-LIMITED GAS FLOW

1. **Perfusion limited** means that _____

_____

_____

_____

2. **Diffusion limited** means that _____

_____

_____

_____

3. Under normal circumstances, the diffusion of oxygen is (circle one):

    a. perfusion limited
    b. diffusion limited
    c. neither perfusion nor diffusion limited

CHAPTER FOUR

PULMONARY FUNCTION MEASUREMENTS

LUNG VOLUMES AND CAPACITIES

1. **Tidal Volume** (V_T) is defined as _____

   _____

   _____

2. **Inspiratory Reserve Volume** (IRV) is defined as _____

   _____

   _____

3. **Expiratory Reserve Volume** (ERV) is defined as _____

   _____

   _____

4. **Residual Volume** (RV) is defined as _____

   _____

   _____

5. **Vital Capacity** (VC) is defined as _____

   _____

   _____

6. **Inspiratory Capacity** (IC) is defined as _____

_____

_____

7. **Functional Residual Capacity** (FRC) is defined as _____

_____

_____

8. **Total Lung Capacity** (TLC) is defined as _____

_____

_____

9. **Residual Volume/Total Lung Capacity Ratio** (RV/TLC $\times$ 100) is defined as _____

_____

_____

10. Compare and contrast the approximate lung volumes and capacities in the average normal male and female between 20 and 30 years of age:

TABLE 4–1 **Approximate Lung Volumes and Capacities in the Average Normal Subject Between 20 and 30 Years of Age**

	MALE		FEMALE	
MEASUREMENT	ml	Approx. % of TLC	ml	Approx. % of TLC
Tidal Volume (V_T)				
Inspiratory Reserve Volume (IRV)				
Expiratory Reserve Volume (ERV)				
Residual Volume (RV)				
Vital Capacity (VC)				
Inspiratory Capacity (IC)				
Functional Residual Capacity (FRC)				
Total Lung Capacity (TLC)				
Residual Volume/Total Lung Capacity Ratio (RV/TLC $\times$ 100)				

11. In an obstructive lung disorder, the _____ , _____ , _____ , and _____ are increased; and the _____ , _____ , _____ and _____ are decreased.

12. In a restrictive lung disorder, the _____ , _____ , _____ , _____ , _____ , and _____ , are all decreased.

PULMONARY MECHANICS

1. **Forced vital capacity** (FVC) is defined as _____

   _____

   _____

   _____

2. **Forced expiratory volume timed** (FEV_T) is defined as _____

   _____

   _____

3. The normal percentage of the total volume exhaled during the following time periods is:

   a. $FEV_{0.5}$ _____ %

   b. $FEV_{1.0}$ _____ %

   c. $FEV_{2.0}$ _____ %

   d. $FEV_{3.0}$ _____ %

4. In obstructive disease, the percentage of FVC that can be forcefully exhaled over a specific period

   of time (_____ increases; _____ decreases; _____ remains the same) .

5. **Forced Expiratory Flow$_{200-1200}$** ($FEF_{200-1200}$) is defined as _____

   _____

   _____

   _____

6. The $FEF_{200-1200}$ is a good index of the (_____ large; _____ small) airway function.

7. **Forced Expiratory Flow$_{25\%-75\%}$** ($FEF_{25\%-75\%}$) is defined as _____

   _____

   _____

   _____

8. The $FEF_{25\%-75\%}$ reflects the status of the _____ to _____ -sized airways.

9. **Peak Expiratory Flow Rate** (PEFR) is defined as _____

_____

_____

10. **Maximum Voluntary Ventilation** (MVV) is defined as _____

_____

_____

11. **Forced Expiratory Volume$_{1\ Second}$/Forced Vital Capacity Ratio** (FEV_1/FVC ratio) is defined as

_____

_____

_____

_____

_____

12. Label the following measurements graphically presented in the **flow-volume loop**:

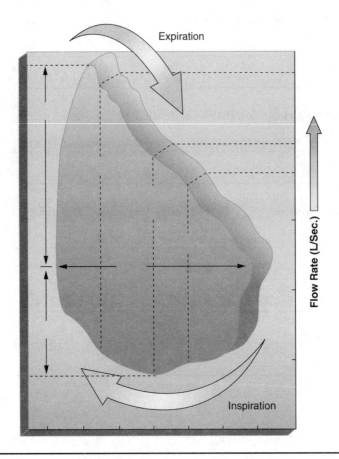

Figure 4–1 *Normal flow-volume loop. PEFR = peak expiration flow rate; PIFR = peak inspiratory flow rate; FVC = forced vital capacity; FEF$_{25\%-75\%}$ = forced expiratory flow$_{25\%-75\%}$; FEF$_{50\%}$ = forced expiratory flow$_{50\%}$ (also called $\dot{V}max_{50}$).*

13. Compare and contrast the following average dynamic flow rate measurements of the healthy male and female between 20 and 30 years of age:

TABLE 4–2 Average Dynamic Flow Rate Measurements of the Healthy Male and Female Between 20 and 30 Years of Age

MEASUREMENT	MALE	FEMALE
FEV_T		
$FEV_{0.5}$		
$FEV_{1.0}$		
$FEV_{2.0}$		
$FEV_{3.0}$		
$FEF_{200-1200}$		
$FEF_{25\%-75\%}$		
PEFR		
MVV		

EFFECTS OF DYNAMIC COMPRESSION ON EXPIRATORY FLOW RATES

1. Approximately the first 30 percent of a forced vital capacity maneuver is effort dependent. **Effort dependent** means that:

2. Approximately the last 70 percent of a forced vital capacity maneuver is effort independent. **Effort independent** means that:

3. The limitation of the flow rate that occurs during the last 70 percent of a forced vital capacity maneuver is due to the _____ of the walls of the airway.

4. As muscular effort and intrapleural pressure increase during a forced expiratory maneuver, the **equal pressure point** moves _____ .

5. Once dynamic compression occurs during a forced expiratory maneuver, increased muscular effort (_____ increases; _____ decreases; _____ has no effect on) airway compression.

CHAPTER FIVE

THE CIRCULATORY SYSTEM

BLOOD

1. List the four major components of blood:

    a. _____

    b. _____

    c. _____

    d. _____

2. The _____ constitute the major portion of the blood cells.

3. In the healthy adult male, there are about _____ million red blood cells in each cubic millimeter of blood.

4. In the healthy adult female, there are about _____ million red blood cells in each cubic millimeter of blood.

5. The percentage of red blood cells in relation to the total blood volume is known as the

    _____ .

6. Compare and contrast the normal hematocrit levels for the following:

    a. Adult male _____ %

    b. Adult female _____ %

    c. Newborn _____ to _____ %

7. Microscopically, the red blood cells appear as biconcave disks, averaging about _____ in diameter and _____ in thickness.

8. The life span of an RBC is about _____ days.

9. The major function of the leukocytes is to _____

_____

_____

_____

_____

10. The normal amount of leukocytes averages between _____ to _____ cells per cubic millimeter of blood.

11. Compare and contrast the normal differential count for the following:

TABLE 5–1 Normal Differential Count

POLYMORPHONUCLEAR GRANULOCYTES	MONONUCLEAR CELLS
Neutrophils	Lymphocytes
Eosinophils	Monocytes
Basophils	

12. The most active leukocytes in response to tissue destruction by bacteria are the _____

_____ .

13. _____ are commonly elevated in response to an allergic condition.

14. _____ are commonly elevated in response to a chronic infection.

15. The _____ are involved in the production of antibodies.

16. Thrombocytes are also called _____ .

17. The normal platelet count in each cubic millimeter of blood ranges between _____

    and _____ .

18. The function of the platelets is to _____

    _____

    _____

    _____

19. Plasma constitutes about _____ percent of the total blood volume.

20. Approximately _____ percent of the plasma consists of water.

21. List the three types of **proteins** found in the plasma:

    a. _____

    b. _____

    c. _____

22. List the **electrolyte cations** found in the plasma:

    a. _____

    b. _____

    c. _____

    d. _____

23. List the **electrolyte anions** found in the plasma:

    a. _____

    b. _____

    c. _____

    d. _____

24. List the four types of **food substances** found in the plasma:

   a. _____

   b. _____

   c. _____

   d. _____

25. List the four types of **waste products** found in the plasma:

   a. _____

   b. _____

   c. _____

   d. _____

THE HEART

1. Label and color the following anatomic structures of the heart:

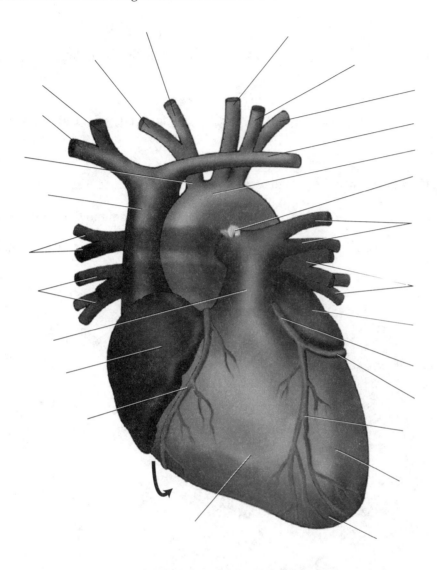

Figure 5–1 *Anterior view of the heart.*

2. The right atrium of the heart receives blood from the _____

_____

3. A one-way valve called the _____ lies between the right atrium and
   right ventricle.

4. The chordae tendineae are secured to the ventricular wall by the _____.

5. Blood leaves the right ventricle through the _____ and enters the right and

   left _____ .

6. After blood passes through the lungs, it returns to the left atrium by way of the _____

   _____ .

7. The bicuspid valve, which lies between the left atrium and left ventricle, is also called the

   _____ .

8. The left ventricle pumps blood through the ascending _____ .

9. The _____ valve prevents the backflow of blood into the left ventricle.

10. Using the following illustration, label the components of the conductive system of the heart:

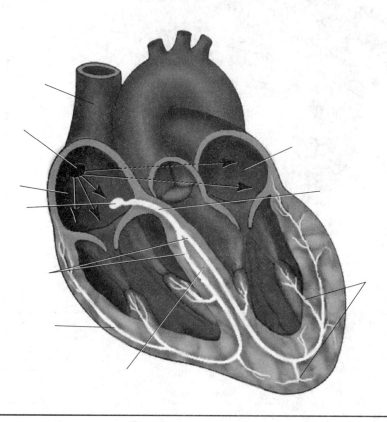

Figure 5–2 *Conductive system of the heart.*

11. The pacemaker of the heart is the _____ .

12. The **cardioaccelerator center** increases heart rate and strength of contraction, by sending _____ _____ impulses to the heart.

13. The **cardioinhibitor center** decreases the heart rate and strength of contraction by sending _____ impulses to the heart.

14. The **P wave** of an electrocardiogram (ECG) represents the _____ _____ .

15. The **QRS complex** represents _____ _____ .

16. The **T wave** represents _____ _____ .

17. Identify the following components of a normal electrocardiogram:

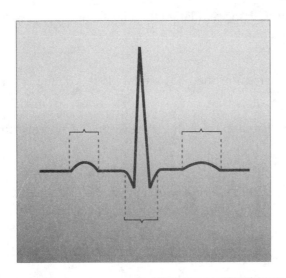

Figure 5–3 *Normal electrocardiogram (ECG) tracing.*

18. The normal adult heart rate is _____ beats per minute.

19. The normal infant heart rate is about _____ beats per minute.

THE PULMONARY AND SYSTEMIC VASCULAR SYSTEMS

1. The pulmonary circulation system begins with the _____ and

   ends in the _____ .

2. The systemic circulation system begins with the _____ and ends

   in the _____ .

3. The arteries are vessels that carry blood (_____ to; _____ away from) the heart.

4. The arteries subdivide into smaller vessels called _____ .

5. The _____ play a major role in the distribution and regulation of blood pressure.

6. Which vessels are referred to as the resistance vessels?

   Answer: _____ .

7. In the capillaries of the pulmonary system, gas exchange is called _____ respiration.

8. In the capillaries of the systemic system, gas exchange is called _____ respiration.

9. Tiny vessels continuous with the capillaries are called _____ .

10. Veins are also known as _____ vessels.

11. Approximately _____ percent of the body's total blood volume is contained within the venous system.

12. The pulmonary arterioles and most of the arterioles in the systemic circulation are controlled by

    _____ impulses.

13. The _____ center, located in the _____ , governs

    the number of _____ impulses sent to the vascular systems.

14. Under normal circumstances, a continual stream of _____ impulses are sent to blood vessels.

15. A moderate state of constant vascular constriction is called _____ .

16. When the vasomotor center is activated to constrict a particular vascular region, it does so by (_____ increasing; _____ decreasing) the number of _____ impulses sent to that vascular area.

17. When the vasomotor center causes vasodilation, it does so by (_____ increasing; _____ decreasing) the number of _____ impulses sent to that vascular region.

18. List the major vascular beds in the systemic system that dilate in response to sympathetic impulses: The arterioles of the:

    a. _____

    b. _____

    c. _____

19. **Baroreceptors**, which are specialized stretch receptors, are also called _____

    _____ .

20. The baroreceptors located in the carotid arteries send neural impulses to the medulla by means of the _____ nerve.

21. The baroreceptors located in the arch of the aorta send neural impulses to the medulla by means of the _____ nerve.

22. When the arterial blood pressure decreases, neural impulses to the medulla (_____ increase; _____ decrease); which, in turn, causes the medulla to (_____ increase; _____ decrease) its sympathetic activity.

23. When the baroreceptors signal the medulla to increase its sympathetic activity, the net result is:

    a. _____

    _____

    b. _____

    _____

    c. _____

    _____

24. In addition to the baroreceptors located in the carotid sinuses and aortic arch, other baroreceptors are found in the:

    a. _____

    b. _____

    c. _____

    d. _____

PRESSURES IN THE PULMONARY AND SYSTEMIC VASCULAR SYSTEMS

1. **Intravascular pressure** is defined as the _____

    _____

    _____

    _____

2. **Transmural pressure** is defined as the _____

    _____

    _____

    _____

3. A positive transmural pressure is when pressure inside the vessel is (_____ greater than; _____ less than; _____ the same as) the pressure outside the vessel.

4. A negative transmural pressure is when the pressure inside the vessel is (_____ greater than; _____ less than; _____ the same as) the pressure outside the vessel.

5. **Driving pressure** is defined as the _____

_____

_____

_____

THE CARDIAC CYCLE AND ITS EFFECT ON BLOOD PRESSURE

1. The maximum pressure generated during ventricular contraction is the _____.

2. When the ventricles relax, the lowest pressure that remains in the arteries prior to the next ventricular contraction is the _____.

3. Compared to the pulmonary circulation, the minimum pressure in the systemic system is about _____ times greater.

4. Using the illustration below, identify the following mean intraluminal blood pressures at various points in the pulmonary and systemic circulation:

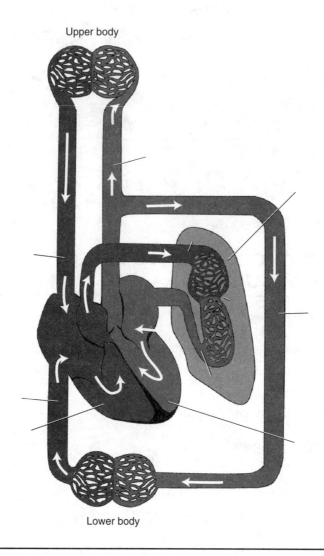

Figure 5–4 *Mean intraluminal blood pressure at various points in the pulmonary and systemic circulation.*

5. Normally, the stroke volume ranges between _____ and _____ .

6. The total volume of blood discharged from the ventricles per minute is called _____

_____ .

7. If an individual has a stroke volume of 55 ml, and a heart rate of 80 beats per minute (beats/min), what is the cardiac output?

   Answer: _____

8. Under normal conditions, when either the stroke volume or heart rate increases, the blood pressure (circle one):

   a. increases
   b. decreases
   c. remains the same

9. The normal adult total blood volume is about _____ liters.

10. In regard to the total blood volume of the normal adults, about _____ percent is in the systemic circulation, _____ percent is in the heart, and _____ percent is in the pulmonary circulation.

11. Overall, about _____ percent of the total blood volume is in the veins, and about _____ percent is in the arteries.

THE DISTRIBUTION OF PULMONARY BLOOD FLOW

1. The fact that blood is **gravity dependent** means that it naturally moves _____

   _____

   _____

   _____

2. The intraluminal pressures in the vessels of the gravity-dependent areas of the lung are (_____ greater than; _____ less than; _____ the same as) the intraluminal pressures in the least gravity-dependent areas.

3. When an individual is in each of the following positions, which part of the lung is the gravity-dependent region?

BODY POSITION	GRAVITY-DEPENDENT LUNG REGION
a. Lying on the back	_____
b. Lying on the stomach	_____
c. Lying on the side	_____
d. Suspended upside down	_____

4. In **zone 1** of the upright lung, the alveolar pressure is sometimes (_____ greater than; _____ less than; _____ the same as) both the arterial and the venous intraluminal pressures.

5. List some conditions that can cause the alveolar pressure to be higher than the arterial and venous pressures:

a. _____

b. _____

c. _____

6. When the alveoli are ventilated but not perfused, _____ is said to exist.

7. In **zone 2** of the upright lung, the arterial intraluminal pressure is (_____ greater than; _____ less than; _____ the same as) the alveolar pressure; and the alveolar pressure is (_____ greater than; _____ less than; _____ the same as) the venous pressure.

8. In **zone 3** of the upright lung, the arterial intraluminal pressure is (_____ greater than; _____ less than; _____ the same as) the alveolar pressure; and the alveolar pressure is (_____ greater than; _____ less than; _____ the same as) the venous pressure.

9. List the three mechanisms that determine stroke volume:

a. _____

b. _____

c. _____

10. **Ventricular preload** refers to _____

_____

_____

11. Within limits, the more myocardial fiber is stretched during diastole, the (_____ more; _____ less) strongly it will contract during systole.

12. **VEDP** stands for _____

13. **VEDV** stands for _____

14. As the VEDV increases the VEDP (circle one):

    a. increases
    b. decreases
    c. remains the same

15. The relationship between the VEDP and cardiac output is known as the _____

_____

16. **Ventricular afterload** is defined as _____

_____

_____

17. Ventricular afterload is determined by:

    a. _____

    _____

    b. _____

    _____

    c. _____

    _____

18. Clinically, what reflects the ventricular afterload the best?

    Answer: _____

19. **Blood pressure** (BP) equals:

    BP = _____ × _____

20. **Myocardial contractility** can be pictured as _____

    _____

    _____

    _____

21. In general, when the contractility of the heart decreases, the cardiac output (circle one):

    a. increases
    b. decreases
    c. remains the same

22. List some clinical assessments that reflect myocardial contractility.

    a. _____

    b. _____

    c. _____

    d. _____

23. An increase in myocardial contractility is referred to as _____

    _____ .

24. A decrease in myocardial contractility is referred to as _____

    _____ .

25. Circulatory resistance is derived as follows:

    Resistance =

26. In general, when the vascular resistance increases, the blood pressure (circle one):

    a. increases
    b. decreases
    c. remains the same

ACTIVE MECHANISMS AFFECTING VASCULAR RESISTANCE

1. Define **active mechanism**: _____

   _____

   _____

   _____

2. In response to a decreased alveolar oxygen pressure, the pulmonary vascular system:

    a. constricts
    b. relaxes
    c. remains the same

3. In response to an increased P_{CO_2} level, the pulmonary vascular system:

    a. constricts
    b. relaxes
    c. remains the same

4. In response to a decreased pH, the pulmonary vascular system:

    a. constricts
    b. relaxes
    c. remains the same

5. In response to an increased H^+ concentration, the pulmonary vascular system:

    a. constricts
    b. relaxes
    c. remains the same

6. List some pharmacologic agents that constrict the pulmonary vessels:

a. _____

b. _____

c. _____

d. _____

e. _____

7. List some pharmacologic agents that relax the pulmonary vessels:

a. _____

b. _____

c. _____

d. _____

8. List some pathologic conditions that increase pulmonary vascular resistance:

a. _____

b. _____

c. _____

d. _____

PASSIVE MECHANISMS AFFECTING VASCULAR RESISTANCE

1. Define **passive mechanism**: _____

_____

_____

_____

2. In response to an increased pulmonary arterial pressure, the pulmonary vascular resistance (circle one):

   a. increases
   b. decreases
   c. remains the same

3. The answer to the above question occurs because of recruitment, which entails _____

   _____

   _____

   and because of distension, which entails _____

   _____

   _____

4. In response to an increased left atrial pressure, the pulmonary vascular resistance (circle one):

   a. increases
   b. decreases
   c. remains the same

5. At high lung volumes, the pulmonary resistance in the alveolar vessels is (_____ high; _____ low).

6. At high lung volumes, the pulmonary resistance in the extra-alveolar vessels is: (_____ high; _____ low).

7. At low lung volumes, the pulmonary resistance in the alveolar vessels is (_____ high; _____ low).

8. At low lung volumes, the pulmonary resistance in the extra-alveolar vessels is: (_____ high; _____ low).

9. At high lung volumes, the pulmonary vascular resistance in the corner vessels is: (_____ high; _____ low).

10. At low lung volumes, the pulmonary vascular resistance in the corner vessels is (_____ high; _____ low).

11. In response to an increased blood volume, pulmonary vascular resistance (circle one):

    a. increases
    b. decreases
    c. remains the same

12. In response to an increased blood viscosity, the pulmonary vascular resistance:

    a. increases
    b. decreases
    c. remains the same

CHAPTER SIX

HEMODYNAMIC MEASUREMENTS

HEMODYNAMIC MEASUREMENTS DIRECTLY OBTAINED BY MEANS OF THE PULMONARY ARTERY CATHETER

1. **Hemodynamic** is defined as _____

   _____

   _____

2. Write the abbreviation and normal range for the following hemodynamic values directly obtained by means of the pulmonary artery catheter:

Table 6–1 **Hemodynamic Values Directly Obtained by Means of the Pulmonary Artery Catheter**

HEMODYNAMIC VALUE	ABBREVIATION	NORMAL RANGE
Central venous pressure		
Right atrial pressure		
Mean pulmonary artery pressure		
Pulmonary capillary wedge pressure (also called pulmonary artery wedge; pulmonary artery occlusion)		
Cardiac output		

HEMODYNAMIC VALUES COMPUTED FROM DIRECT MEASUREMENTS

1. Write the abbreviation and normal range for the following computed hemodynamic values:

Table 6–2 Computed Hemodynamic Values

HEMODYNAMIC VARIABLE	ABBREVIATION	NORMAL RANGE
Stroke volume		
Stroke volume index		
Cardiac index		
Right ventricular stroke work index		
Left ventricular stroke work index		
Pulmonary vascular resistance		
Systemic vascular resistance		

2. **Stroke volume** (SV) is defined as _____

_____

_____

3. List the major determinants of stroke volume:

   a. _____

   b. _____

   c. _____

4. Complete the following equation:

   SV =

5. If a patient has a cardiac output of 5.5 L/min and a heart rate of 87 beats/min, what is the stroke volume?

Answer: _____

6. The **stroke volume index** (SVI) is derived by_____

_____

_____

7. If a patient has a stroke volume of 55 ml and a body surface area of 2.5 m2, what is the SVI?

Answer: _____

8. Clinically, what does the SVI reflect?

a. _____

b. _____

c. _____

9. The **cardiac index** (CI) is calculated by_____

_____

_____

10. If a patient has a cardiac output of 7 L/min and a body surface area of 2.5 m2, what is the CI?

    Answer: _____

11. What does the **right ventricular stroke work index** (RVSWI) measure?

    _____

    _____

    _____

12. Clinically, what does the RVSWI reflect?

    _____

    _____

13. Complete the following equation:

    RVSWI =

14. If a patient has a SVI of 40 ml, a $\overline{PA}$ of 25 mm Hg, and a CVP of 10 mm Hg, what is the RVSWI?

    Answer: _____

15. What does the **left ventricular stroke work index** (LVSWI) measure?

_____

_____

_____

16. Clinically, what does the LVSWI reflect?

_____

_____

17. Complete the following equation:

    LVSWI =

18. If a patient has an SVI of 45 ml, an MAP of 125 mm Hg, and a PCWP of 10 mm Hg, what is the LVSWI?

    Answer: _____

19. Fill in factors that increase and decrease the following hemodynamic variables:

Table 6–3 **Factors Increasing and Decreasing Stroke Volume (SV), Stroke Volume Index (SVI), Cardiac Output (CO), Cardiac Index (CI), Right Ventricular Stroke Work Index (RVSWI), and Left Ventricular Stroke Work Index (LVSWI)**

INCREASES	DECREASES
Positive Inotropic Drugs (Increased Contractility)	**Negative Inotropic Drugs (Decreased Contractility)**
Abnormal Conditions	**Abnormal Conditions**
	Hyperinflation of Lungs

20. The pulmonary vascular system is a (_____ high; _____ low) resistance system.

21. The systemic vascular system is a (_____ high; _____ low) resistance system.

22. Clinically, what does **pulmonary vascular resistance** (PVR) indicate?

    Answer: _____

23. Complete the following equation:

    PVR =

24. If a patient has a $\overline{PA}$ of 20, a PCWP of 10 mm Hg, and a CO of 7 L/min, what is the PVR?

Answer: _____

25. Fill in under each category below the factors that increase pulmonary vascular resistance:

Table 6–4   **Factors that Increase Pulmonary Vascular Resistance (PVR)**

CHEMICAL STIMULI   **PATHOLOGIC FACTORS**

PHARMACOLOGIC AGENTS

HYPERINFLATION OF LUNGS

HUMORAL SUBSTANCES

---

26. Fill in under the categories below factors that decrease pulmonary vascular resistance (PVR):

Table 6–5   Factors that Decrease Pulmonary Vascular Resistance (PVR)

PHARMACOLOGIC AGENTS	HUMORAL SUBSTANCES

27. Clinically, what does **systemic vascular resistance** (SVR) indicate?

    Answer: _____

28. Complete the following equation:

    SVR =

29. If a patient has an MAP of 105 mm Hg, a CVP of 10 mm Hg, and a CO of 6 L/min, what is the SVR?

    Answer: _____

30. Fill in under the categories below factors that increase and decrease systemic vascular resistance (SVR):

Table 6–6   **Factors that Increase and Decrease Systemic Vascular Resistance (SVR)**

INCREASES	DECREASES
Vasoconstricting Agents	**Vasodilating Agents**
Abnormal Conditions	**Abnormal Conditions**

CHAPTER SEVEN

OXYGEN TRANSPORT

OXYGEN TRANSPORT

1. Compare and contrast the normal ranges for the following blood gas values:

Table 7–1 **Normal Blood Gas Values Ranges**

BLOOD GAS VALUE	ARTERIAL	VENOUS
pH		
P_{CO_2}		
HCO_3^-		
P_{O_2}		

2. The term **dissolved** means that when a gas like oxygen enters the plasma, it _____

_____

_____

_____

3. Clinically, which portion of the oxygen transport system is measured to assess the patient's partial pressure of oxygen (P_{O_2})?

Answer: _____

4. Complete the following exercise:

   a. If an individual has an arterial oxygen partial pressure (Pa_{O_2}) of 50 mm Hg, about how many ml of oxygen are dissolved in every 100 ml of blood?

   Answer: _____ ml O_2/100 ml of blood

   b. In regard to the above answer, what is the vol% of dissolved oxygen?

   Answer: _____

5. Vol% (volumes percent) is defined as _____

   _____

6. Each red blood cell (RBC) contains approximately _____ million hemoglobin molecules.

7. The normal adult hemoglobin is designated as Hb _____ .

8. In the normal adult hemoglobin, how many heme group(s) are there?

   Answer: _____

9. Write the reversible reaction of O_2 with Hb:

10. When two oxygen molecules are bound to one Hb molecule, the Hb is said to be _____ percent saturated with oxygen; an Hb molecule with one oxygen molecule is _____ percent saturated.

11. Hemoglobin bound with oxygen is called _____ .

12. Hemoglobin not bound with oxygen is called _____

    or _____ .

13. The amount of oxygen bound to hemoglobin is (_____ indirectly; _____ directly) related to the partial pressure of oxygen.

14. The **globin portion** of each hemoglobin molecule consists of _____

    _____

    _____

    _____

15. **Fetal hemoglobin** (HbF) has _____ chains and _____ chains.

16. Hemoglobin changed from the ferrous state to the ferric state is known as _____

    _____ .

17. Compare and contrast the normal hemoglobin values for the following:

    a. Adult male: _____ g% Hb

    b. Adult female: _____ g% Hb

    c. Average infant: _____ g% Hb

18. Hemoglobin constitutes about _____ percent of the RBC weight.

19. Each gram percent (g%) Hb is capable of carrying about _____ ml of oxygen.

20. At a normal arterial oxygen pressure (Pa_{O_2}) the hemoglobin saturation (Sa_{O_2}) is only 97 percent because of the following normal physiologic shunts:

    a. _____

    _____

    b. _____

    _____

    c. _____

    _____

21. Complete the following total oxygen transport exercises:

Case A

A 23-year-old female with severe asthma presents with the following clinical data:

Hb: 13 g%
Pa_{O_2}: 55 mm Hg
Sa_{O_2}: 85%
Cardiac output: 6 L/min

a. How much dissolved O_2 is the patient transporting in every 100 ml of blood?

Answer: _____ ml O_2/100 ml blood (vol%)

b. How much O_2 is bound to the hemoglobin in every 100 ml of blood?

Answer: _____ ml O_2/100 ml blood (vol%)

c. What is the total O_2 content of the arterial blood (Ca_{O_2})?

Answer: Ca_{O_2} = _____ (vol% O_2; or ml O_2/100 ml blood)

d. Since the Ca_{O_2} is in reference to 1/10 of 1 liter of blood, how many ml of O_2 are available for tissue metabolism in one liter of blood?

Answer: _____ ml O_2/liter

e. Since this patient has a cardiac output of 6 L/min, how many ml of O_2 are available for tissue metabolism in 1 minute?

Answer: _____ ml O_2/min

Case B

A 62-year-old male with severe emphysema presents with the following clinical data:

- Hb: 18 g%
- Pa_{O_2}: 50 mm Hg
- Sa_{O_2}: 80%
- Cardiac output: 3.5 L/min
- $P\bar{v}_{O_2}$: 25 mm Hg
- $S\bar{v}_{O_2}$: 50%
- PA_{O_2}: 150 mm Hg

a. How much dissolved O_2 is the patient transporting in every 100 ml of blood?

   Answer: _____ ml O_2/100 ml blood (vol%)

b. How much O_2 is bound to the hemoglobin in every 100 ml of blood?

   Answer: _____ ml O_2/100 ml blood (vol% O_2)

c. What is the total O_2 content of the arterial blood (Ca_{O_2})?

   Answer: Ca_{O_2} = _____ (vol% O_2; or ml O_2/100 ml blood)

d. Since the Ca_{O_2} is in reference to 1/10 of 1 liter of blood, how many ml of O_2 are available for tissue metabolism in 1 liter of blood?

   Answer: _____ ml O_2/liter

e. Since this patient has a cardiac output of 3.5 L/min, how many ml of O_2 are available for tissue metabolism in 1 minute?

   Answer: _____ ml O_2/min

f. What is the patient's total oxygen content of mixed venous blood ($C\bar{v}_{O_2}$)?

Answer: $C\bar{v}_{O_2}$ = _____ (vol% O_2; or ml O_2/100 ml blood)

g. What is the patient's total oxygen content of capillary blood (Cc_{O_2})?

Answer: Cc_{O_2} = _____ (vol% O_2; or ml O_2/100 ml blood)

OXYGEN DISSOCIATION CURVE

1. The **oxygen dissociation curve** illustrates the _____ of hemoglobin that is

chemically bound to oxygen at each oxygen _____ .

2. Clinically, the **flat portion** of the oxygen dissociation curve is significant because it illustrates that

a. _____

_____

b. _____

_____

c. _____

_____

3. Clinically, the **steep portion** of the oxygen dissociation curve is significant because it illustrates that

a. _____

_____

_____

b. _____

_____

4. Using the oxygen dissociation curve nomogram below, answer the next two questions (a. and b.).

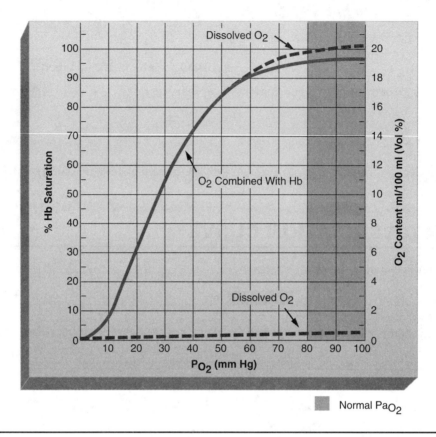

Figure 7–1 *Oxygen dissociation curve.*

a. If the P_{O_2} is 50 mm Hg, what is the percentage of hemoglobin that is bound to oxygen?

Answer: _____

b. What is the oxygen content level in vol%?

Answer: _____

5. The P_{50} represents _____

_____

_____

6. Normally, the P_{50} is about ————————————— mm Hg.

7. When the oxygen dissociation curve shifts to the right, the P_{50} (circle one):

    a. increases
    b. decreases
    c. remains the same

8. When the oxygen dissociation curve shifts to the left, the P_{50} (circle one):

    a. increases
    b. decreases
    c. remains the same

9. List factors that shift the oxygen dissociation curve to the

    a. left: ———————————————————

    ———————————————————

    ———————————————————

    ———————————————————

    ———————————————————

    ———————————————————

    b. right: ———————————————————

    ———————————————————

    ———————————————————

    ———————————————————

10. Clinically, when the oxygen dissociation curve shifts to the *right*, the loading of oxygen in the lungs at any given P_{O_2} (circle one):

    a. increases
    b. decreases
    c. remains the same

11. Clinically, when the oxygen dissociation curve shifts to the *right*, the plasma P_{O_2} reduction necessary to unload oxygen at the tissue sites is:

    a. less than normal
    b. greater than normal
    c. the same as normal

12. Clinically, when the oxygen dissociation curve shifts to the *left*, the loading of oxygen in the lungs at any given P_{O_2}:

    a. increases
    b. decreases
    c. remains the same

13. Clinically, when the oxygen dissociation curve shifts to the *left*, the plasma P_{O_2} reduction necessary to unload oxygen at the tissue sites is:

    a. less than normal
    b. greater than normal
    c. the same as normal

OXYGEN TRANSPORT STUDIES

1. List the most common oxygen transport studies performed in the clinical setting:

    a. _____

    b. _____

    c. _____

    d. _____

    e. _____

    f. _____

2. **Total oxygen delivery** to the peripheral tissues is dependent on the:

    a. _____

    b. _____

    c. _____

3. Complete the following formula:

    $\dot{D}_{O_2} =$

4. If a patient has a cardiac output of 3.5 L/min and a Ca_{O_2} of 12 vol%, what is the total amount of oxygen delivered to the patient's peripheral cells?

Answer: _____

5. List three conditions that reduce an individual's total oxygen delivery:

a. _____

b. _____

c. _____

6. The **arterial-venous content difference** $[C(a - v)_{O_2}]$ is defined as the difference _____

_____

_____

7. Complete the following formula:

$$C(a - \bar{v})_{O_2} =$$

8. If a patient has a Ca_{O_2} of 13 vol% and a $C\bar{v}_{O_2}$ of 9 vol%, what is the patient's $C(a - \bar{v})_{O_2}$?

Answer: _____

9. List some clinical factors that *increase* the $C(a - \bar{v})_{O_2}$:

a. _____

b. _____

    1. _____

    2. _____

    3. _____

    4. _____

10. List some clinical factors that *decrease* the $C(a - \bar{v})_{O_2}$:

a. _____

b. _____

c. _____

d. _____

e. _____

11. The amount of oxygen extracted by the peripheral tissues during the period of one minute is

called _____ or _____ .

12. Complete the following formula:

$$\dot{V}_{O_2} =$$

13. If a patient has a cardiac output of 7.5 L/min and a $C(a - \bar{v})_{O_2}$ of 8 vol%, what is the patient's $\dot{V}_{O_2}$?

Answer: _____

14. List some clinical factors that *increase* the $\dot{V}_{O_2}$:

    a. _____

    b. _____

    c. _____

    d. _____

15. List some clinical factors that *decrease* the $\dot{V}_{O_2}$:

    a. _____

    b. _____

    c. _____

    d. _____

16. An individual's oxygen consumption index is derived by dividing the $\dot{V}_{O_2}$ by the _____

    _____

17. The average oxygen consumption index ranges between _____ and _____ ml O_2/m^2.

18. The oxygen extraction ratio (O_2ER) is defined as the amount of oxygen

    _____

    _____

    _____

    _____

19. The O_2ER is also known as the

    a. _____

    b. _____

20. Complete the following formula:

    $O_2ER =$

21. The normal O_2ER is _____ percent.

22. a. If a patient has a Ca_{O_2} of 14 vol%, and a $C\bar{v}_{O_2}$ of 7 vol%, what is the patient's O_2ER?

    Answer: _____ percent

    b. If the above patient has a total oxygen delivery of 850 ml/minute, then this would mean that

    during a course of 1 minute, _____ ml of oxygen are metabolized by the tissues and

    _____ ml of oxygen are returned to the lungs.

23. List some clinical factors that *increase* the O_2ER:

    a. _____

    b. _____

       1. _____

       2. _____

       3. _____

       4. _____

    c. _____

    d. _____

24. List some clinical factors that *decrease* the O_2ER:

    a. _____

    b. _____

    c. _____

    d. _____

    e. _____

    f. _____

25. The normal $S\bar{v}_{O_2}$ is —————— percent.

26. Clinically, an $S\bar{v}_{O_2}$ of about —————— percent is acceptable.

27. List some clinical factors that *decrease* the $S\bar{v}_{O_2}$:

    a. _____

    b. _____

      1. _____

      2. _____

      3. _____

      4. _____

28. A reduction in the $S\bar{v}_{O_2}$ indicates that the $C(a - \bar{v})_{O_2}$, $\dot{V}_{O_2}$, and O_2ER are (circle one):

    a. increasing
    b. decreasing
    c. remaining the same

29. List some clinical factors that *increase* the $S\bar{v}_{O_2}$:

    a. _____

    b. _____

    c. _____

    d. _____

    e. _____

30. An increase in the $S\bar{v}_{O_2}$ indicates that the $C(a - \bar{v})_{O_2}$, $\dot{V}_{O_2}$, and O_2ER are (circle one):

    a. increasing
    b. decreasing
    c. remaining the same

31. Indicate with the following code system how the clinical factors listed will likely alter a patient's total oxygen delivery, $\dot{V}_{O_2}$, $C(a - \bar{v})_{O_2}$, O_2ER, and $S\bar{v}_{O_2}$.

Code system: same = unchanged status; $\uparrow$ = increase; = $\downarrow$ decrease

Table 7–2 Clinical Factors Affecting Various Oxygen Transport Study Values

CLINICAL FACTORS	OXYGEN TRANSPORT STUDIES				
	D_{O_2} (1000 ml O_2/min)	$\dot{V}_{O_2}$ (250 ml O_2/min)	$C(a - \bar{v})_{O_2}$ (5 vol%)	O_2ER (25%)	$S\bar{v}_{O_2}$ (75%)
$\uparrow O_2$ Consumption					
$\downarrow O_2$ Consumption					
$\downarrow$ Cardiac Output					
$\uparrow$ Cardiac Output					
$\downarrow Pa_{O_2}$					
$\uparrow Pa_{O_2}$					
$\downarrow$ Hb					
$\uparrow$ Hb					
Peripheral Shunting					

$\uparrow$: increase; $\downarrow$: decrease.

MECHANISMS OF PULMONARY SHUNTING

1. **Pulmonary shunting** is defined as _____

   _____

   _____

   _____

   _____

   _____

   _____

   _____

   _____

2. List the two major categories of conditions that cause a **true shunt mechanism**:

   a. _____

   b. _____

3. An **anatomic shunt** exists when _____

   _____

   _____

   _____

4. The normal anatomic shunt is about _____ to _____ percent.

5. List three common causes of **anatomic shunting**:

   a. _____

   b. _____

   c. _____

6. List three common causes of **capillary shunting**:

   a. _____

   b. _____

   c. _____

7. The sum of the anatomic and capillary shunts is referred to as _____ or

   _____ .

8. What does **refractory** to oxygen therapy mean? _____

   _____

   _____

   _____

   _____

   _____

9. A **shunt-like effect** is said to exist when _____

   _____

   _____

10. List some common causes of the shunt-like effect mechanism:

   a. _____

   b. _____

   c. _____

11. What is **venous admixture**? _____

   _____

   _____

   _____

12. Complete the following shunt equation:

$$\frac{\dot{Q}s}{\dot{Q}\tau} =$$

13. A 42-year-old female is on a volume-cycled mechanical ventilator on a day when the barometric pressure is 740 mm Hg. The patient is receiving an FI_{O_2} of 0.45. The following clinical data are obtained:

 Hb: 10 g%
 Pa_{O_2}: 65 mm Hg (Sa_{O_2} = 91%)
 Pa_{CO_2}: 35 mm Hg
 $P\bar{v}_{O_2}$: 30 mm Hg ($S\bar{v}_{O_2}$ = 60%)

Using the information above, calculate the patient's PA_{O_2}, Cc_{O_2}, Ca_{O_2}, and $C\bar{v}_{O_2}$.

a. PA_{O_2} =

 Answer: ⎯⎯⎯⎯⎯⎯⎯⎯⎯⎯⎯

b. Cc_{O_2} =

 Answer: ⎯⎯⎯⎯⎯⎯⎯⎯⎯⎯⎯

c. Ca_{O_2} =

 Answer: ⎯⎯⎯⎯⎯⎯⎯⎯⎯⎯⎯

d. $C\bar{v}_{O_2} =$

Answer: _____

e. Using the clinical data above, calculate the patient's pulmonary shunt:

$$\frac{\dot{Q}s}{\dot{Q}T} =$$

Answer: _____

14. What is the clinical significance of the following calculated shunts:

a. below 10 percent: _____

_____

b. 10–20 percent: _____

_____

c. 20–30 percent: _____

_____

d. greater than 30 percent: _____

_____

15. List three clinical factors that cause the calculation of pulmonary shunting to be unreliable:

a. _____

b. _____

c. _____

TISSUE HYPOXIA

1. **Hypoxic hypoxia** is defined as _____

   _____

   _____

2. List some conditions that can cause hypoxic hypoxia:

   a. _____

   b. _____

   c. _____

3. **Anemic hypoxia** is defined as _____

   _____

   _____

   _____

4. List two conditions that cause anemic hypoxia:

   a. _____

   _____

   b. _____

   _____

5. **Circulatory hypoxia** is defined as _____

   _____

   _____

   _____

   _____

6. List two major forms of circulatory hypoxia:

   a. _____

   b. _____

7. **Histotoxic hypoxia** is defined as _____

   _____

   _____

8. Define **cyanosis:** _____

   _____

   _____

   _____

9. Define **polycythemia:** _____

   _____

   _____

CHAPTER EIGHT

CARBON DIOXIDE TRANSPORT AND ACID-BASE BALANCE

CARBON DIOXIDE TRANSPORT

1. List the three ways that carbon dioxide is transported from the tissue cells to the lungs in the **plasma**:

   a. _____

   b. _____

   c. _____

2. List the three ways that carbon dioxide is transported from the tissue cells to the lungs in the **red blood cells**:

   a. _____

   b. _____

   c. _____

3. In what form is most of the carbon dioxide carried to the lungs?

   Answer: _____

4. The answer to the above question accounts for about _____ percent of the total amount of carbon dioxide transported to the lungs.

5. Using the following illustration, write the various chemical reaction(s) carbon dioxide goes through at the tissue sites to be transported to the lungs.

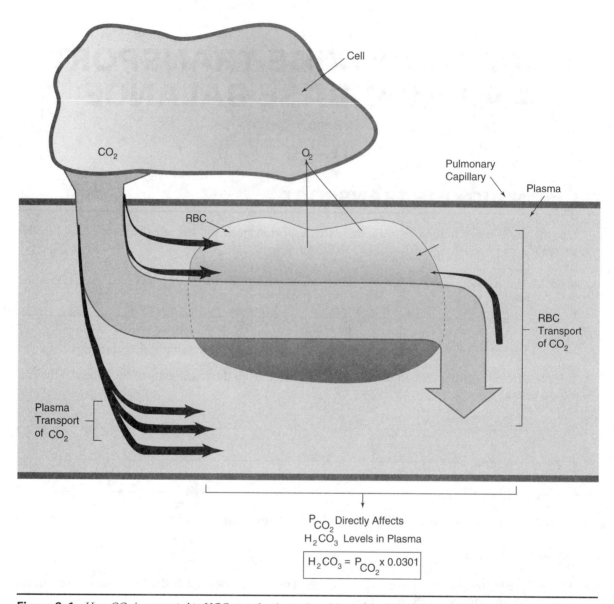

Figure 8–1 *How CO_2 is converted to HCO_3^- at the tissue sites. Most of the CO_2 that is produced at the tissue cells is carried to the lungs in the form of HCO_3^-.*

6. Unlike the S-shaped oxygen dissociation curve, the carbon dioxide curve is much more _____

_____.

CARBON DIOXIDE ELIMINATION AT THE LUNGS

1. Using the following carbon dioxide dissociation curve nomogram, if the P_{CO_2} increases from 25 mm Hg to 40 mm Hg, the carbon dioxide content increases from _____ vol% to _____ vol%.

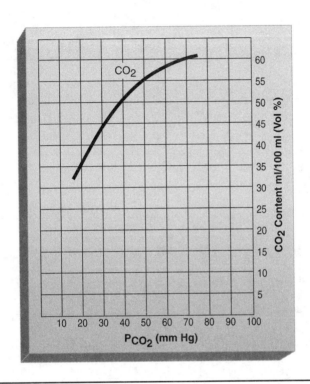

Figure 8–2 *Carbon dioxide dissociation curve.*

CARBON DIOXIDE DISSOCIATION CURVE AND ACID-BASE BALANCE

1. The fact that deoxygenated blood enhances the loading of carbon dioxide is called the _____

_____.

2. **Electrolytes** are _____

_____

_____

3. A **buffer** is a _____

_____

_____

_____

4. A **strong acid** is an acid that _____

_____

_____

5. A **weak acid** is an acid that _____

_____

_____

6. A **strong base** is a base that _____

_____

_____

7. A **weak base** is a base that _____

_____

_____

8. A **dissociation constant** refers to _____

_____

_____

_____

9. In the equation below, circle the portion of the acid or base system that is in the *dissociated state*:

$$HA \rightleftharpoons [H^+] + [A^-]$$

10. A pH of 7 is _____ .

11. A pH *less* than 7 is_____ .

12. A pH *greater* than 7 is _____ .

13. In chemistry, the pH is defined as _____

_____

_____

14. The above definition of pH is written as:

pH =

15. A pH of 7 is equal to _____ mole/L.

16. An *acid* is a substance that (_____ accepts; _____ donates) [H$^+$].

17. An *acid* is a substance that (_____ increases; _____ decreases) the numerical value of the pH.

18. A *base* is a substance that (_____ accepts; _____ donates) [H$^+$].

19. A *base* is a substance that (_____ increases; _____ decreases) the numerical value of the pH.

20. List the three mechanisms that maintain the narrow pH range:

a. _____

_____

b. _____

_____

c. _____

_____

21. The most important buffer system in respiratory physiology is the _____

_____ combination.

22. The **Henderson-Hasselbalch equation** uses the components of the $H_2CO_3^-/HCO_3^-$ system in the following way:

    pH =

23. **pK** is derived from _____

    _____

    _____

24. Normally, the pK is _____ .

25. The normal HCO_3^- to $H_2CO_3^-$ ratio is _____ to _____ .

26. An HCO_3^- to $H_2CO_3^-$ ratio of 17 : 1 means the pH is (circle one):

    a. normal
    b. less than normal
    c. greater than normal

27. An HCO_3^- to H_2CO_3 ratio of 26 : 1 means the pH is:

    a. normal
    b. less than normal
    c. greater than normal

THE ROLE OF THE P_{CO_2}/HCO_3^-/pH RELATIONSHIP IN ACID-BASE BALANCE

1. During acute ventilatory failure (hypoventilation), the blood (check one):

    a. P_{CO_2} (_____ increases; _____ decreases; _____ remains the same)

    b. H_2CO_3 (_____ increases; _____ decreases; _____ remains the same)

    c. HCO_3^- (_____ increases; _____ decreases; _____ remains the same)

    d. HCO_3^- to H_2CO_3 ratio (_____ increases; _____ decreases; _____ remains the same)

    e. pH (_____ increases; _____ decreases; _____ remains the same)

2. In chronic ventilatory failure, the kidneys work to correct the pH status by (circle one):

    a. excreting HCO_3^-
    b. retaining H_2CO_3
    c. excreting H_2CO_3
    d. retaining $H_2CO_3^-$

3. In chronic ventilatory failure, partial or complete renal compensation can be verified when the HCO_3^- and pH readings on the $P_{CO_2}/HCO_3^-/pH$ nomogram are:

    a. greater than expected for a particular Pa_{CO_2}
    b. less than expected for a particular Pa_{CO_2}

4. During **acute alveolar hyperventilation** the blood (check one):

    a. P_{CO_2} (_____ increases; _____ decreases; _____ remains the same)

    b. H_2CO_3 (_____ increases; _____ decreases; _____ remains the same)

    c. HCO_3^- (_____ increases; _____ decreases; _____ remains the same)

    d. HCO_3^- to H_2CO_3 ratio (_____ increases; _____ decreases; _____ remains the same)

    e. pH (_____ increases; _____ decreases; _____ remains the same)

5. In **chronic alveolar hyperventilation**, the kidneys work to correct the pH status by:

    a. excreting HCO_3^-
    b. retaining H_2CO_3
    c. excreting H_2CO_3
    d. retaining HCO_3^-

6. In chronic alveolar hyperventilation, partial or complete renal compensation can be verified when the HCO_3^- and pH readings are (circle one):

    a. greater than expected for a particular Pa_{CO_2}
    b. less than expected for a particular Pa_{CO_2}

7. True ____ False ____   As a general rule, the kidneys have a tendency to overcompensate for an abnormal pH.

8. When **metabolic acidosis** is present, the HCO_3^- and pH readings are (circle one):

    a. greater than expected for a particular Pa_{CO_2}
    b. less than expected for a particular Pa_{CO_2}

9. List three common causes of metabolic acidosis:

    a. _____

    b. _____

    c. _____

10. In response to a metabolic acidosis condition, the ventilatory rate (circle one):

    a. increases
    b. decreases
    c. remains the same

11. When **metabolic alkalosis** is present, the HCO_3^- and pH readings are:

    a. greater than expected for a particular Pa_{CO_2}
    b. less than expected for a particular Pa_{CO_2}

12. List five common causes of metabolic alkalosis:

    a. _____

    b. _____

    c. _____

    d. _____

    e. _____

13. Using the P_{CO_2}/HCO_3^-/pH nomogram below, answer the next four questions (a.–d.):

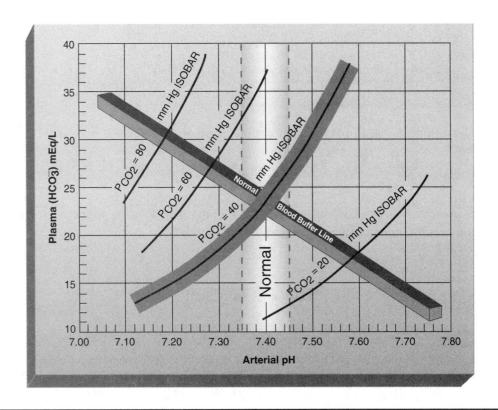

Figure 8–3 *Nomogram of P_{CO_2}/HCO_3^-/pH relationship.*

a. If a patient's ventilatory rate suddenly decreased, and the patient's Pa_{CO_2} increased to 70 mm Hg, what changes would be expected in the pH and HCO_3^- level?

Answer: pH _____

   HCO_3^- _____

b. If a patient's ventilatory rate suddenly increased, causing the patient's Pa_{CO_2} to decrease to 20 mm Hg, what would be the expected pH and HCO_3^- changes?

Answer: pH _____

   HCO_3^- _____

c. If a patient presents with a pH of 7.2 and a Pa_{CO_2} of 60 mm Hg, does the patient have a metabolic or respiratory acid-base imbalance, or a combination of both?

Answer: _____

Which does the above patient have, a base excess or a base deficit?

Answer: _____

In order to return the patient's pH back to 7.4, how much of a base excess or base deficit does the patient have?

Answer: _____

d. If a patient presents with a pH of 7.52 and a Pa_{CO_2} of 25 mm Hg, does the patient have a metabolic or respiratory acid-base imbalance, or a combination of both?

Answer: _____

Which does the patient have, a base excess or a base deficit?

Answer: _____

In order to return the patient's pH back to 7.4, how much of a base excess or base deficit does the patient have?

Answer: _____

CHAPTER NINE

VENTILATION-PERFUSION RELATIONSHIPS

VENTILATION-PERFUSION RATIO

1. The normal alveolar ventilation is about _____ L/min.

2. The normal pulmonary capillary blood flow is about _____ L/min.

3. The average overall ventilation/perfusion ratio is _____ to _____, or _____.

4. In the normal individual in the upright position, the $\dot{V}/\dot{Q}$ ratio in the upper lung region is (_____ higher; _____ lower) than 0.8.

5. In the normal individual in the upright position, the $\dot{V}/\dot{Q}$ ratio in the lower lung region is (_____ higher; _____ lower) than 0.8.

6. In the upright lung, the $\dot{V}/\dot{Q}$ ratio progressively (_____ increases; _____ decreases; _____ remains the same) from the top to the bottom.

7. The $P_{A_{O_2}}$ is determined by the balance between

   a. _____

   _____

   b. _____

   _____

8. The PA_{CO_2} is determined by the balance between

   a. _____

   _____

   b. _____

   _____

9. When the $\dot{V}/\dot{Q}$ ratio increases, the PA_{CO_2} decreases because _____

   _____

   _____

   _____

10. When the $\dot{V}/\dot{Q}$ ratio increases, the PA_{O_2} decreases because _____

    _____

    _____

    _____

    _____

11. In the upright lung, an increased $\dot{V}/\dot{Q}$ ratio is found in the (circle one):

    a. upper lung regions
    b. middle lung regions
    c. lower lung regions

12. When the $\dot{V}/\dot{Q}$ ratio decreases, the PA_{O_2} decreases because _____

    _____

    _____

    _____

13. When the $\dot{V}/\dot{Q}$ ratio decreases, the PA_{CO_2} increases because _____

    _____

    _____

    _____

14. In the upright lung, a decreased $\dot{V}/\dot{Q}$ ratio is found in the (circle one):

    a. upper lung regions
    b. middle lung regions
    c. lower lung regions

15. In the upright lung, the Pc_{O_2} (_____ increases; _____ decreases; _____ remains the same) from the top to the bottom.

16. In the upright lung, the Pc_{CO_2} (_____ increases; _____ decreases; _____ remains the same) from the top to the bottom.

17. In the upright lung, the pH in the end-capillary blood (_____ increases; _____ decreases; _____ remains the same) from the top to the bottom.

18. **Internal respiration** is defined as _____

    _____

    _____

19. Normally, about _____ ml of oxygen are consumed by the tissue cells in 1 minute.

20. Normally, the tissue cells produce about _____ ml of carbon dioxide in 1 minute.

21. **Respiratory quotient** (RQ) is defined as the _____

    _____

    _____

22. The respiratory quotient is expressed as:

    RQ =

23. **External respiration** is defined as _____

    _____

    _____

24. **Respiratory exchange ratio** (RR) is defined as the _____

_____

_____

25. List some pulmonary disorders that increase the $\dot{V}/\dot{Q}$ ratio:

   a. _____

   _____

   b. _____

   _____

   c. _____

   _____

   d. _____

   _____

   e. _____

   _____

26. List some pulmonary disorders that decrease the $\dot{V}/\dot{Q}$ ratio:

   a. _____

   _____

   b. _____

   _____

   c. _____

   _____

CHAPTER TEN

CONTROL OF VENTILATION

THE RESPIRATORY COMPONENTS OF THE MEDULLA

1. It is now believed that the DRG and VRG neurons in the medulla oblongata are responsible for coordinating the intrinsic rhythmicity of respiration. DRG and VRG are abbreviations for

   a. DRG: _____

   a. VRG: _____

2. The DRG consists chiefly of (circle one):

   a. inspiratory neurons
   b. expiratory neurons
   c. inspiratory and expiratory neurons

3. The VRG consist of:

   a. inspiratory neurons
   b. expiratory neurons
   c. inspiratory and expiratory neurons

4. Which of the following is activated only during heavy exercise or stress?

   a. DRG
   b. VRG

5. Where is the **apneustic center** located? _____

   _____

   _____

6. If unrestrained, the apneustic center causes (circle one):

   a. prolonged expiration
   b. prolonged inspiration

7. Which of the following suppress(es) the function of the apneustic center (circle one)?

   a. DRG
   b. pneumotaxic center
   c. VRG

MONITORING SYSTEMS THAT INFLUENCE THE RESPIRATORY COMPONENTS OF THE MEDULLA

1. The respiratory components (DRG and VRG) of the medulla are primarily influenced by an excessive concentration of _____.

2. Where are the **central chemoreceptors** located?_____

   _____

   _____

3. The **blood–brain barrier** is very permeable to _____ molecules, and relatively impermeable to _____ and _____ ions.

4. Write the chemical reaction that forms carbonic acid when CO_2 moves into the cerebrospinal fluid:

   $CO_2 +$

5. How do the central chemoreceptors respond to the liberated hydrogen ions [H+] produced in the above reaction?

   _____

   _____

   _____

   _____

6. In essence, the central chemoreceptors regulate ventilation through the (_____ direct; _____ indirect) effects of CO_2 on the _____ .

7. The **peripheral chemoreceptors** are _____

   _____

   _____

   _____

8. Where are the peripheral chemoreceptors located? _____

   _____

   _____

   _____

9. When activated by a low Pa_{O_2}, the carotid bodies send neural impulses to the respiratory components of the medulla by way of the _____ nerve; the aortic bodies send neural impulses to the medulla by way of the _____ nerve.

10. Which of the following play a greater role in causing the ventilatory rate to increase in response to a decreased Pa_{O_2} (circle one)?

    a. carotid bodies
    b. aortic bodies

11. At about what Pa_{O_2} level are the peripheral chemoreceptors significantly activated?

    Answer: _____

12. Suppression of the peripheral chemoreceptors is seen when the Pa_{O_2} falls below _____

    _____ .

13. Why are the peripheral chemoreceptors totally responsible for the control of ventilation when the Pa_{CO_2} level is chronically high?

_____

_____

_____

_____

_____

_____

_____

14. In response to a chronically high CO_2 level, the sensitivity of the peripheral chemoreceptors (circle one):

    a. increases
    b. decreases
    c. remains the same

15. List some clinical conditions in which the P_{O_2} is normal, but the oxygen content is dangerously low:

    a. _____

    b. _____

    c. _____

16. List some other factors that stimulate the peripheral chemoreceptors:

    a. _____

    b. _____

    c. _____

    d. _____

    e. _____

17. In addition to an increase in ventilation, list some other responses that occur when the peripheral chemoreceptors are stimulated:

a. _____

b. _____

c. _____

d. _____

e. _____

REFLEXES THAT INFLUENCE VENTILATION

1. What activates the **Hering-Breuer reflex?**_____

_____

2. When activated, the Hering-Breuer reflex cause(s) _____

_____

3. What activates the **deflation reflex?**_____

_____

4. When activated, the deflation reflex cause(s) _____

_____

5. What activates the **irritant reflex?**_____

_____

_____

6. Where are the irritant receptors located? _____

_____

7. When activated, the irritant reflex cause(s) _____

_____

8. Where are the **J receptors** located?_____

_____

9. What activates the J receptors?

   a. _____

   b. _____

   c. _____

   d. _____

   e. _____

   f. _____

10. When activated, the J receptors cause _____

_____

11. In response to an elevated systemic blood pressure, the **aortic and carotid sinus baroreceptors**

    cause _____

_____

12. In response to a reduced systemic blood pressure, the aortic and carotid sinus baroreceptors cause

_____

_____

13. How do the following stimuli affect ventilation?

    a. A sudden cold stimulus _____

    _____

    _____

    b. A sudden pain _____

    _____

    _____

c. Irritation of the pharynx or larynx _____

_____

_____

_____

d. Stretching of the anal sphincter _____

_____

_____

e. Light pressure applied to the thorax _____

_____

_____

CHAPTER ELEVEN

CARDIOPULMONARY PHYSIOLOGY OF THE FETUS AND THE NEWBORN

FETAL LUNG DEVELOPMENT

1. List the four periods of lung development during fetal life.

   a. _____

   b. _____

   c. _____

   d. _____

2. The lungs first appear as a small bud arising from the esophagus on the _____ day of embryonic life.

3. By the 16th week of gestation, there are about _____ generations of bronchial airways.

4. By the _____ week of gestation, the air–blood interface between the alveoli and the pulmonary capillaries and the quantity of pulmonary surfactant are usually sufficient to support life.

PLACENTA

1. Anatomically, the placenta consists of about 15 to 20 segments called _____ .

2. Label and color the following anatomic structures of the placenta:

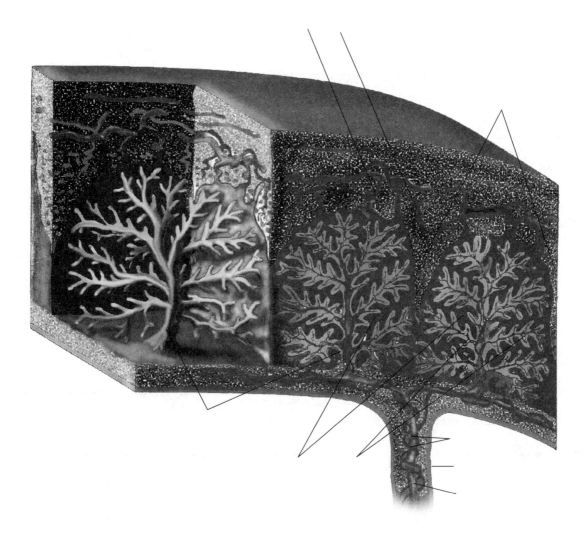

Figure 11–1 *Anatomic structure of the cotyledon of the placenta.*

3. Deoxygenated blood is carried from the fetus to the placenta by way of two _____

   _____ .

4. Normally, the P_{O_2} in the umbilical arteries is about _____ mm Hg and the P_{CO_2} is about

   _____ mm Hg.

5. Explain why the maternal blood P_{CO_2} is frequently lower than expected during the last trimester of pregnancy.

_____

_____

_____

_____

6. Once in the intervillous space, oxygen transfers from the maternal to fetal blood because of the

a. _____

_____

b. _____

_____

c. _____

_____

7. As oxygenated fetal blood flows out of the chorionic villi, the P_{O_2} is about _____ mm Hg, and the

P_{CO_2} is about _____ mm Hg.

8. Oxygenated fetal blood flows out of the chorionic villi and returns to the fetus by way of the _____

_____ .

9. List the three factors thought to be responsible for the wide variance between the maternal and fetal P_{O_2} and P_{CO_2}.

a. _____

_____

b. _____

_____

c. _____

_____

FETAL CIRCULATION

1. As oxygenated blood from the placenta returns to the fetus, about one-half of the blood enters the liver of the fetus and the rest enters the inferior vena cava by flowing through the _____ _____ .

2. Once in the right atrium of the fetus, most of the blood flows directly into the left atrium through the _____ .

3. The blood in the left atrium of the fetus enters the _____ and is then pumped primarily to the _____ and _____ .

4. Most of the fetal blood that passes into the pulmonary artery from the right ventricle bypasses the lungs by passing through the _____ and flows directly into the _____ _____ .

5. Approximately _____ percent of the fetal circulation passes through the lungs and returns to the left atrium via the _____ .

6. The Pa_{O_2} in the descending aorta is about _____ mm Hg.

Matching:

7. Directions: In *Column A*, match the order (i.e., from first to last) in which fetal blood passes through the structures in *Column B*.

COLUMN A	COLUMN B
Order	**Structure**
_____	a. common iliac arteries
_____	b. external and internal iliacs
_____	c. ductus arteriosus
_____	d. umbilical arteries
_____	e. ductus venosus

8. Describe the changes the special structures of the fetal circulation go through after birth:

   a. _____

   _____

   _____

   b. _____

   _____

   _____

   c. _____

   _____

   _____

   d. _____

   _____

   _____

   e. _____

   _____

   _____

   f. _____

   _____

   _____

9. Describe the three primary mechanisms that remove the fluid from the fetal lungs during the first 24 hours of life:

   a. _____

   _____

   _____

   b. _____

   _____

   _____

   c. _____

   _____

   _____

10. About _____ million primitive alveoli are present at birth.

11. The number of alveoli continues to increase until about _____ years of age.

BIRTH

1. List some of the stimuli that cause the infant to take its first breath at birth:

   a. _____

   b. _____

   c. _____

2. During the first breath, it is estimated that the infant's intrapleural pressure decreases to about

   _____ cm H_2O before any air enters the lungs.

3. About _____ ml of air enters the lungs during the first breath.

4. The average lung compliance (C_L) of the newborn is about _____ .

5. The average airway resistance (R_{aw}) of the newborn is about _____ .

6. List the two major mechanisms that account for the decreased pulmonary vascular resistance when an infant inhales for the first time:

a. _____

_____

_____

b. _____

_____

_____

7. Describe the mechanism that causes the foramen ovale to close functionally at birth:

_____

_____

_____

_____

_____

_____

_____

8. At birth, the newborn's P_{O_2} must increase to more than _____ to _____ mm Hg in order for the ductus arteriosus to close.

9. Describe the meaning of persistent pulmonary hypertension of the neonate (PPHN):

_____

_____

_____

_____

10. Persistent pulmonary hypertension of the neonate was previously known as _____

_____ .

11. List other substances that are released at birth that are believed to contribute to the constriction of the ductus arteriosus:

    a. _____

    b. _____

    c. _____

CONTROL OF VENTILATION IN THE NEWBORN

1. Although inhibited during fetal life, the _____ and _____

   _____ chemoreceptors play a major role in activating the first breath at

   birth.

2. Stimulation of the newborn's trigeminal nerve causes the infant's respiration and heart rate to

   _____ .

3. Stimulation of the preterm infant's irritant reflex is commonly followed by _____

   _____ .

4. Stimulation of the term infant's irritant reflex causes _____

   _____ .

5. The head paradoxical reflex is: _____

   _____ .

NORMAL CLINICAL PARAMETERS IN THE NEWBORN

1. Compare and contrast the approximate lung volumes and capacities of the newborn:

TABLE 11–1 Approximate Lung Volumes and Capacities of the Newborn

Tidal volume (V_T)   Vital capacity (VC)
Residual volume (RV)   Functional residual capacity (FRC)
Expiratory reserve volume (ERV)   Inspiratory capacity (IC)
Inspiratory reserve volume (IRV)   Total lung capacity (TLC)

---

2. Write the normal vital sign ranges of the newborn:

TABLE 11–2 Normal Vital Sign Ranges of the Newborn

Respiratory rate (RR)
Heart rate (HR)
Blood pressure (BP)

CHAPTER TWELVE

RENAL FAILURE AND ITS EFFECTS ON THE CARDIOPULMONARY SYSTEM

THE KIDNEYS

1. Label and color the following structures that form the **kidney**:

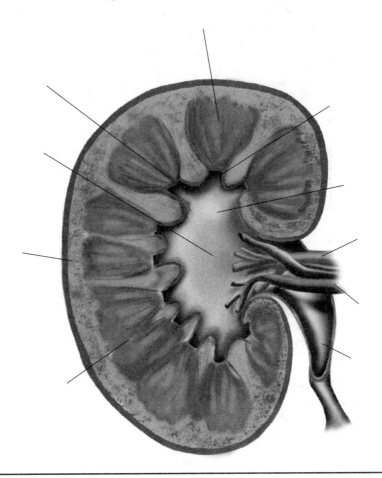

Figure 12–1 *Cross-section of the kidney.*

2. Label and color the following structures of the **nephron**:

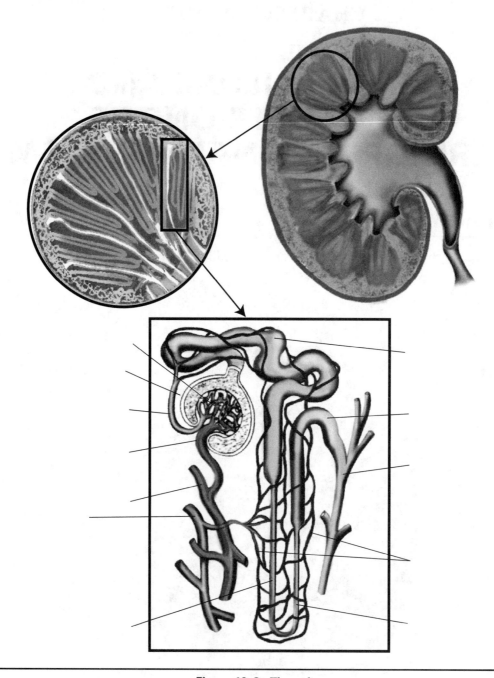

Figure 12–2   *The nephron.*

3. Label and color the following **blood vessels** of the kidney:

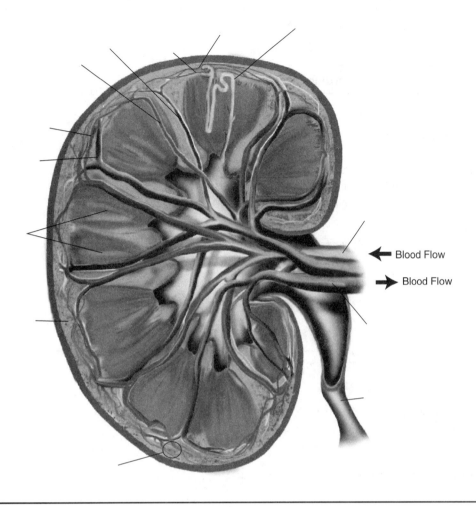

Blood Flow

Blood Flow

Figure 12–3 *Blood vessels of the kidney.*

URINE FORMATION

1. Compare and contrast the forces of glomerular filtration:

TABLE 12–1   Forces of Glomerular Filtration

FACTORS	FORCE
Enhances Filtration	
Glomerular capillary blood pressure	
Opposes Filtration	
Fluid pressure in Bowman's capsule	
Osmotic force (caused by the protein concentration difference)	_____
Net Filtration Pressure	

2. List the three major structures responsible for tubular reabsorption:

    a. _____

    b. _____

    c. _____

3. The bulk of **tubular reabsorption** occurs in the _____

    _____ .

4. **Tubular secretion** is the mechanism by which _____

    _____

    _____

    _____

    _____

5. The most important substances transported into the tubules by means of secretion are

    _____ and _____ ions.

URINE CONCENTRATION AND VOLUME

1. The kidneys control the concentration and volume of urine by virtue of the following two mechanisms:

   a. _____

   b. _____

   _____

2. The **juxtamedullary nephrons** are located deep into the _____

   _____ .

3. The normal osmolality of the glomerular filtrate is approximately _____ mOsm/L.

4. The osmolality of the interstitial fluid ranges from about _____ mOsm/L in the cortex to

   about _____ mOsm/L as the juxtamedullary nephron descends into the renal medulla.

5. ADH is produced in the _____ and released by the

   _____ .

6. When the atrial blood volume and pressure increase, the production of ADH (circle one):

   a. increases
   b. decreases
   c. remains the same

7. When the atrial blood volume and pressure decrease, the production of ADH:

   a. increases
   b. decreases
   c. remains the same

8. When the production of ADH decreases, the volume of urine (_____ increases; _____ decreases).

9. When the production of ADH increases, the volume of urine (_____ increases; _____ decreases).

10. The urine produced by the healthy kidney has a specific gravity of about _____ to

    _____ .

REGULATION OF ELECTROLYTE CONCENTRATION

1. List some of the more important ions regulated by the kidneys:

   a. _____

   b. _____

   c. _____

2. When the extracellular fluid becomes too acidic, the kidneys excrete _____ ions into the urine.

3. When the extracellular fluid becomes too alkaline, the kidneys excrete (primarily) _____

   _____ into the urine.

4. The two major mechanisms responsible for maintaining an individual's blood volume at a consistent level are

   a. _____

   b. _____

RENAL FAILURE

1. List some congenital renal disorders:

   a. _____

   b. _____

   c. _____

2. Urinary tract infections are seen more often in (_____ men; _____ women).

3. List some factors that predispose an individual to urinary flow obstruction:

   a. _____

   b. _____

   c. _____

   d. _____

   e. _____

4. List some causes of kidney inflammation:

   a. _____

   b. _____

   c. _____

5. Name the form of cancer that accounts for about 70 percent of all cancers of early childhood.

   Answer: _____ .

6. List some common prerenal causes of renal failure:

   a. _____

   b. _____

   c. _____

   d. _____

7. What is one of the early clinical manifestations of **prerenal failure**?

   Answer: _____ .

8. List the five categories of **renal** abnormalities that cause renal failure:

   a. _____

   b. _____

   c. _____

   d. _____

   e. _____

9. List some **postrenal** abnormalities that cause renal failure:

   a. _____

   b. _____

10. Positive pressure ventilation (_____ increases; _____ decreases) urinary output.

11. Negative pressure ventilation (_____ increases; _____ decreases) urinary output.

12. When positive pressure ventilation causes the blood volume and, therefore, the pressure in the atria to decrease, the release of ADH (circle one):

   a. increases
   b. decreases
   c. remains the same

13. When the concentration of ADH increases, the amount of urine formed:

   a. increases
   b. decreases
   c. remains the same

CARDIOPULMONARY PROBLEMS CAUSED BY RENAL FAILURE

1. Hypertension and edema develop in renal failure because of the kidney's inability to excrete

   _____ .

2. When the kidneys fail, metabolic acidosis develops because the following changes occur:

   a. H^+ (_____ increases; _____ decreases)

   b. K^+ (_____ increases; _____ decreases)

   c. HCO_3^- (_____ increases; _____ decreases)

3. **Hypochloremia** causes (circle one):
   a. acidosis
   b. alkalosis

4. **Hypokalemia** causes:
   a. acidosis
   b. alkalosis

5. **Hyperchloremia** causes:
   a. acidosis
   b. alkalosis

6. **Hyperkalemia** causes:
   a. acidosis
   b. alkalosis

7. Which two mechanisms contribute to the anemia seen in chronic renal failure?

   a. _____

   _____

   _____

   _____

   b. _____

   _____

   _____

   _____

8. Why do patients with chronic renal failure have a tendency to bleed?

_____

_____

_____

9. Why is pericarditis seen in about 50% of persons with chronic renal failure?

_____

_____

_____

_____

_____

CHAPTER THIRTEEN

AGING AND ITS EFFECTS ON THE CARDIOPULMONARY SYSTEM

THE INFLUENCE OF AGING ON THE RESPIRATORY SYSTEM

1. The growth and development of the lungs is essentially complete by about _____ years of age.

2. Most of the pulmonary function indices reach their maximum level between _____ and _____ years of age.

3. With aging, the elastic recoil of the lungs (_____ increases; _____ decreases; _____ remains the same), and the lung compliance (_____ increases; _____ decreases; _____ remains the same),

4. With aging, identify which changes occur (check one) with the following lung volumes and capacities:

   a. RV (_____ increases; _____ decreases; _____ remains the same)

   b. IC (_____ increases; _____ decreases; _____ remains the same)

   c. IC (_____ increases; _____ decreases; _____ remains the same)

   d. TLC (_____ increases; _____ decreases; _____ remains the same)

   e. RV/TLC (_____ increases; _____ decreases; _____ remains the same)

   f. FRC (_____ increases; _____ decreases; _____ remains the same)

   g. ERV (_____ increases; _____ decreases; _____ remains the same)

5. With aging, identify which changes occur with the following dynamic maneuvers of ventilation:

   a. FVC (_____ increases; _____ decreases; _____ remains the same)

   b. PEFR (_____ increases; _____ decreases; _____ remains the same)

   c. FEF$_{25\%-75\%}$ (_____ increases; _____ decreases; _____ remains the same)

   d. FEV$_1$ (_____ increases; _____ decreases; _____ remains the same)

   e. FEV$_1$/FVC ratio (_____ increases; _____ decreases; _____ remains the same)

   f. FRC (_____ increases; _____ decreases; _____ remains the same)

   g. MVV (_____ increases; _____ decreases; _____ remains the same)

6. With aging, identify which changes occur with the following components of the respiratory system:

   a. Pulmonary diffusing capacity (_____ increases; _____ decreases; _____ remains the same)

   b. Alveolar deadspace ventilation (_____ increases; _____ decreases; _____ remains the same)

   c. P(A − a)$_{O_2}$ (_____ increases; _____ decreases; _____ remains the same)

   d. Pa$_{O_2}$ (_____ increases; _____ decreases; _____ remains the same)

   e. Pa$_{CO_2}$ (_____ increases; _____ decreases; _____ remains the same)

   f. HCO$_3^-$ (_____ increases; _____ decreases; _____ remains the same)

   g. pH (_____ increases; _____ decreases; _____ remains the same)

   h. C(a − v̄)$_{O_2}$ (_____ increases; _____ decreases; _____ remains the same)

   i. Hemoglobin concentration (_____ increases; _____ decreases; _____ remains the same)

ARTERIAL BLOOD GASES

1. With aging, the ventilatory response to both hypoxia and hypercapnia (circle one):

   a. increases
   b. decreases
   c. remains the same

2. With aging, the maximal oxygen uptake ($\dot{V}_{O_2}$ max):

   a. increases
   b. decreases
   c. remains the same

THE INFLUENCE OF AGING ON THE CARDIOVASCULAR SYSTEM

1. With aging, the elasticity of the heart:

   a. increases
   b. decreases
   c. remains the same

2. With aging, the work of the heart:

   a. increases
   b. decreases
   c. remains the same

3. With aging, the heart rate reacts as follows in response to stress:

   a. is more likely to increase dramatically
   b. is less likely to increase dramatically
   c. remains the same

4. What is the maximum heart rate for a 70-year-old?

   Answer: _____

5. With aging, identify which changes develop (check one) with the following components of the cardiovascular system:

   a. Stroke volume (_____ increases; _____ decreases; _____ remains the same)

   b. Cardiac output (_____ increases; _____ decreases; _____ remains the same)

   c. Resting pulse pressure (_____ increases; _____ decreases; _____ remains the same)

   d. Systolic blood pressure (_____ increases; _____ decreases; _____ remains the same)

   e. Peripheral vascular resistance (_____ increases; _____ decreases; _____ remains the same)

CHAPTER FOURTEEN

EXERCISE AND ITS EFFECTS ON THE CARDIOPULMONARY SYSTEM

EFFECTS OF EXERCISE

1. During heavy exercise

   a. Alveolar ventilation may increase as much as _____-fold.

   b. Oxygen diffusion capacity may increase as much as _____-fold.

   c. Cardiac output may increase as much as _____-fold.

   d. Muscle blood flow may increase as much as _____-fold.

   e. Oxygen consumption may increase as much as _____-fold.

   f. Heat production may increase as much as _____-fold.

2. Muscle training can increase muscle size and strength _____ to _____ percent.

3. The efficiency of intracellular metabolism may increase by _____ to _____ percent.

4. The size of the heart chambers and the heart mass of well-trained athletes may be increased by _____ percent.

5. The point at which anaerobic metabolism develops is called _____ .

VENTILATION

1. It has been suggested that the increased ventilation seen in exercise is caused by:

   a. _____

   _____

   _____

   b. _____

   _____

   _____

   c. _____

   _____

   _____

2. During strenuous exercise, an adult alveolar ventilation can increase to (circle one):
   a. 40 L/min
   b. 60 L/min
   c. 80 L/min
   d. 100 L/min
   e. 120 L/min

3. During exercise, the increased alveolar ventilation is caused mainly by an increased _____ of ventilation, rather than an increased _____ of ventilation.

4. During very heavy exercise, both an increased _____ and _____ of ventilation is seen.

5. During very heavy exercise, the tidal volume is usually about what percent (circle one) of the vital capacity?
   a. 10%
   b. 20%
   c. 30%
   d. 40%
   e. 50%

6. There are three distinct consecutive breathing patterns seen during mild and moderate exercise.

   a. The first stage is characterized by _____

   _____

   _____

   _____

   b. The second stage is typified by _____

   _____

   _____

   _____

   c. During the third stage, _____

   _____

   _____

   _____

7. The maximum alveolar ventilation generated during heavy exercise under normal conditions is

   about _____ to _____ percent of the maximum voluntary ventilation.

8. At rest, normal oxygen consumption ($\dot{V}_{O_2}$) is about _____ ml per minute.

9. During exercise, the skeletal muscles may account for more than _____ percent of the ($\dot{V}_{O_2}$).

10. The Pa_{O_2} remains constant during:
    I. mild exercise
    II. moderate exercise
    III. heavy exercise

       a. I only
       b. I and II only
       c. I, II, and III only

11. It has been shown that the increased oxygen diffusion capacity results from the _____

    _____ during exercise.

12. During exercise, the $P(A - a)_{O_2}$ remains essentially constant until what percent (circle one) of the maximal oxygen consumption is reached?

    a. 10%
    b. 20%
    c. 30%
    d. 40%
    e. 50%

CIRCULATION

1. These essential physiologic responses must occur in order for the circulatory system to supply the working muscles with an adequate amount of blood:

    a. _____

    b. _____

    c. _____

2. The two circulatory effects of the sympathetic discharge are

    a. _____

       _____

       _____

       _____

    b. _____

       _____

       _____

       _____

3. The increased oxygen demands during exercise are met almost entirely by _____

    _____ .

4. The increased cardiac output during exercise results from

   a. _____

   b. _____

   c. _____

5. The increased stroke volume during exercise is primarily due to _____ in the working muscles.

6. The ability of the heart to accommodate the increased venous return and, subsequently, increase cardiac output is due to the _____ mechanism.

7. The maximum heart rate for a 55-year-old is about _____ .

8. When the stroke volume decreases, the heart rate (_____ increases; _____ decreases; _____ remains the same), and when the stroke volume increases, the heart rate (_____ increases; _____ decreases; _____ remains the same).

9. The stroke volume is influenced by

   a. _____

   _____

   b. _____

   _____

   c. _____

   _____

10. The body's ability to increase the heart rate and stroke volume during exercise progressively (_____ increases; _____ decreases) with age.

11. There is almost always an increase in arterial blood pressure during exercise because

a. _____

_____

_____

b. _____

_____

_____

c. _____

_____

_____

12. As oxygen consumption and cardiac output increase during exercise, the pulmonary:

a. Systolic pressure (_____ increases; _____ decreases; _____ remains the same)

b. Diastolic pressure (_____ increases; _____ decreases; _____ remains the same)

c. Arterial (mean) pressure (_____ increases; _____ decreases; _____ remains the same)

d. Wedge pressure (_____ increases; _____ decreases; _____ remains the same)

13. The dilation of the blood vessels in the working muscles is caused primarily by _____

_____ acting on the arterioles.

STROKE VOLUME VERSUS HEART RATE IN INCREASING THE CARDIAC OUTPUT

1. During very heavy exercise, the increased _____ accounts for a much greater pro-

portion of the increased cardiac output than the _____ .

2. The stroke volume reaches its maximum when the maximum cardiac output is only at approxi-

mately _____ percent.

3. After the stroke volume reaches its maximum, any further increase in cardiac output is solely due

   to an _____ .

4. Maximum exercise taxes the respiratory system only about _____ percent of maximum.

BODY TEMPERATURE/CUTANEOUS
BLOOD FLOW RELATIONSHIP

1. List the symptoms that, collectively, are referred to as heat stroke:

   _____

   _____

   _____

   _____

   _____

   _____

2. The primary treatment of heat stroke consists of

   a. _____

      _____

   b. _____

      _____

   c. _____

      _____

   d. _____

      _____

CARDIOVASCULAR REHABILITATION

1. List the four phrase(s) of the cardiovascular rehabilitation process:

   a. Phase I: _____

   _____

   b. Phase II: _____

   _____

   c. Phase III: _____

   _____

   d. Phase IV: _____

   _____

CHAPTER FIFTEEN

HIGH ALTITUDE AND ITS EFFECTS ON THE CARDIOPULMONARY SYSTEM

EFFECTS OF HIGH ALTITUDE

1. The barometric pressure is about half the sea level value of 760 mm Hg at an altitude of _____ feet.

2. One of the most prominent features of acclimatization is _____

_____

3. In lowlanders who ascend to high altitudes, the RBCs increase for about _____ before the production rate levels off.

4. People who live at high altitudes commonly demonstrate (circle one):

   a. mild respiratory acidosis
   b. normal arterial blood gas values
   c. mild respiratory alkalosis

5. The oxygen diffusion capacity of lowlanders who are acclimatized to high altitude:

   a. increases
   b. decreases
   c. remains the same

6. The oxygen diffusion capacity of high-altitudes natives is about _____ than predicted.

7. At high altitude, the alveolar-arterial P_{O_2} difference $[P(A - a)_{O_2}]$ (circle one):

   a. increases
   b. decreases
   c. remains the same

8. At high altitude, the overall ventilation-perfusion ratio improves in response to the (_____ increased; _____ decreased) pulmonary arterial blood pressure.

9. In individuals, who have acclimatized to high altitude, and in high-altitude natives, cardiac output (circle one):

   a. increases
   b. decreases
   c. remains the same

10. As an individual ascends, the pulmonary vascular system:

    a. constricts
    b. dilates
    c. remains the same

OTHER PHYSIOLOGIC CHANGES

1. In high-altitude natives, the concentration of myoglobin in skeletal muscles (circle one):

   a. increases
   b. decreases
   c. remains the same

2. Acute mountain sickness is characterized by _____

   _____

   _____

   _____

3. The symptoms of acute mountain sickness are generally most severe on the _____

   _____

   _____

4. Although the exact cause of high-altitude pulmonary edema is not fully understood, it may be associated with pulmonary (_____ vasoconstriction; _____ vasodilation), and with a/an (_____ increased; _____ decreased) permeability of the pulmonary capillaries.

5. High-altitude cerebral edema is characterized by_____

_____

_____

_____

6. Chronic mountain sickness is characterized by_____

_____

_____

_____

CHAPTER SIXTEEN

HIGH-PRESSURE ENVIRONMENTS AND THEIR EFFECT ON THE CARDIOPULMONARY SYSTEM

DIVING

1. For every 33 feet below the water surface, the pressure increases _____ .

2. a. If an individual fully inhales to a total lung capacity of 5.5 liters at sea level, and dives to a depth of 99 feet, the lungs will be compressed to about:

   Answer: _____

   b. What is the pressure within the above diver's lungs?

   Answer: _____

3. The maximum time of a breath-hold dive is a function of

    a. _____

    _____

    b. _____

    _____

4. In regard to the P_{CO_2}, the so-called respiratory drive "breaking point" is about _____ mm Hg.

5. The so-called CO_2 paradox occurs as a diver (_____ descends; _____ ascends) and the O_2 paradox

    occurs as the diver (_____ descends; _____ ascends).

6. The fall in $P_{A_{O_2}}$ as a diver returns to the surface is known as the _____

    _____ .

7. The dive response consists of

    a. _____

    b. _____

    c. _____

8. List some of the signs and symptoms collectively referred to as decompression sickness:

    a. _____

    b. _____

    c. _____

    d. _____

    e. _____

HYPERBARIC MEDICINE

1. Identify indications for hyperbaric oxygenation for the following clinical conditions:

TABLE 16–1   Indications for Hyperbaric Oxygenation

GAS DISEASES

VASCULAR INSUFFICIENCY STATES

INFECTIONS

DEFECTS IN OXYGEN TRANSPORT

---

2. Hyperbaric oxygen is effective in the treatment of carbon monoxide poisoning. The administration of hyperbaric oxygen

a. _____

_____

_____

_____

b. _____

_____

_____

_____

c. _____

_____

_____

_____

3. Breathing 100-percent oxygen at one atmosphere changes the Hb_{CO} half-life, to less than _____

_____ .

ANSWERS

The question numbers refer to the questions in this workbook. The reference numbers refer to pages in the textbook, *Cardiopulmonary Anatomy and Physiology: Essentials for Respiratory Care*, 3rd edition.

CHAPTER ONE

THE ANATOMY OF THE RESPIRATORY SYSTEM

ANSWERS

THE UPPER AIRWAY

1. (ref. pg. 6)
2. a. to act as a conductor of air
   b. to prevent foreign materials from entering the tracheobronchial tree
   c. serve as an important area involved in speech and smell (ref. pg. 5)
3. a. filter
   b. humidify (ref. pg. 5)
   c. warm
4. (ref. pg. 7)
5. (ref. pg. 7)
6. pseudostratified ciliated columnar (ref. pg. 6)
7. a. superior nasal turbinates
   b. middle nasal turbinates
   c. inferior nasal turbinates (ref. pg. 6)
8. (ref. pg. 9)
9. levator veli platinum (ref. pg. 10)
10. stratified squamous (ref. pg. 10)
11. palatoglossal, palatopharyngeal (ref. pg. 10)
12. pseudostratified ciliated columnar (ref. pg. 11)
13. eustachian tube (ref. pg. 11)
14. stratified squamous (ref. pg. 11)
15. stratified squamous (ref. pg. 11)
16. (ref. pg. 10)

THE LOWER AIRWAYS

1. a. acts as a passageway of air between the pharynx and the trachea
   b. works as a protective mechanism against the aspiration of solid and liquids
   c. generates sounds for speech (ref. pg. 11)

2. (ref. pg. 12)
3. (ref. pg. 14)
4. vocal ligament (ref. pg. 13)
5. thyroid cartilage (ref. pg. 13)
6. rima glottidis or glottis (ref. pg. 13)
7. stratified squamous (ref. pg. 13)
8. pseudostratified ciliated columnar (ref. pg. 13)
9. Valsalva's maneuver (ref. pg. 15)
10. (ref. pg. 15)
11. (ref. pg. 16)

THE TRACHEOBRONCHIAL TREE

1. (ref. pg. 17)
2. a. epithelial lining
   b. lamina propria
   c. cartilaginous layer (ref. pg. 18)
3. pseudostratified ciliated columnar (ref. pg. 18)
4. submucosal glands (ref. pg. 19)
5. sol layer, gel layer (ref. pg. 19)
6. (ref. pg. 19)
7. a. cigarette smoke
   b. dehydration
   c. positive pressure ventilation
   d. endotracheal suctioning
   e. high inspired oxygen concentration
   f. hypoxia
   g. atmospheric pollutants
   h. general anesthetics
   i. parasympatholytics (ref. pg. 20)
8. a. histamine
   b. heparin
   c. slow-reacting substance of anaphylaxis
   d. platelet-activating factor
   e. eosinophilic chemotactic factors of anaphylaxis (ref. pg. 21)
9. 11 to 13, 1.5 to 2.5 (ref. pg. 23)
10. carina (ref. pg. 23)
11. 25, 40 to 60 (ref. pg. 23)
12. terminal bronchioles (ref. pg. 28)
13. increases (ref. pg. 25)
14. terminal bronchioles (ref. pg. 26)
15. mediastinal lymph nodes, the pulmonary nerves, muscular pulmonary arteries and veins, a portion of the esophagus, some visceral pleura (ref. pg. 26)
16. azygos, hemiazygos, intercostal veins (ref. pg. 27)
17. bronchopulmonary anastomoses (ref. pg. 27)

THE SITES OF GAS EXCHANGE

1. a. respiratory
   b. alveolar
   c. alveolar (ref. pg. 27)
2. (ref. pg. 28)
3. (ref. pg. 29)
4. 300 (ref. pg. 28)
5. 70 (ref. pg. 28)
6. respiratory bronchioles, alveolar ducts, and alveolar clusters (ref. pg. 28)
7. 130,000 (ref. pg. 28)
8. a. acinus
   b. terminal respiratory unit
   c. lung parenchyma
   d. functional units (ref. pg. 28)
9. squamous pneumocyte (ref. pg. 28)
10. granular pneumocyte (ref. pg. 28)
11. 95% (ref. pg. 29)
12. type II (ref. pg.29)
13. pores of Kohn (ref. pg. 29)
14. alveolar macrophages (ref. pg. 30)
15. tight space, loose space (ref. pgs. 30–31)

PULMONARY VASCULAR SYSTEM AND LYMPHATIC SYSTEM

1. (ref. pg. 33)
2. resistance (ref. pg. 32)
3. 0.1 μ, 10 μ (ref. pg. 32)
4. capacitance (ref. pg. 34)
5. visceral pleura (ref. pg. 34)
6. loose space of the interstitium (ref. pg. 34)
7. (ref. pg. 36)

NEURAL CONTROL OF THE LUNGS

1. autonomic nervous system (ref. pg. 37)
2. (ref. pg. 37)
3. epinephrine or norepinephrine (ref. pg. 37)
4. relax (ref. pg. 37)
5. constrict (ref. pg. 37)
6. acetylcholine (ref. pg. 37)

THE LUNGS

1. first (ref. pg. 38)
2. sixth, eleventh (ref. pg. 38)
3. hilum (ref. pg. 38)
4. costal, mediastinal (ref. pg.38)
5. oblique fissure, fourth (ref. pg. 38)
6. costal, mediastinal (ref. pg. 38)
7. (ref. pg. 38)
8. (ref. pg. 39)
9. (ref. pg. 40)
10. (ref. pg. 41)

THE MEDIASTINUM, PLEURAL MEMBRANES, AND THORAX

1. trachea, heart, major blood vessels, various nerves, portions of the esophagus, thymus gland, and lymph nodes (ref. pg. 41)
2. visceral (ref. pg. 41)
3. parietal (ref. pg. 41)
4. pleural cavity (ref. pg. 41)
5. a. manubrium sterni
   b. the body
   c. xiphoid process (ref. pg. 42)
6. true ribs (ref. pg. 43)
7. false (ref. pg. 43)
8. floating (ref. pg. 48)
9. (ref. pg. 42)
10. (ref. pg. 43)

THE DIAPHRAGM

1. central tendon (ref. pg. 44)
2. esophagus, aorta, several nerves, and the inferior vena cava (ref. pg. 44)
3. phrenic (ref. pg. 44)
4. first, second (ref. pg. 45)
5. sternum (ref. pg. 46)
6. chest, anteroposterior (ref. pg. 46)
7. scapula, shoulders, arms (ref. pg. 47)
8. upward, outward (ref. pg. 49)
9. (ref. pg. 50)
10. downward, inward (ref. pg. 52)

CHAPTER TWO

VENTILATION

ANSWERS

PRESSURE DIFFERENCES ACROSS THE LUNGS

1. driving pressure (ref. pg. 58)
2. transairway pressure (ref. pg. 59)
3. transpulmonary pressure (ref. pg. 59)
4. transthoracic pressure (ref. pg. 60)
5. 5 mm Hg (ref. pg. 58)
6. 7 mm Hg (ref. pg. 59)
7. 4 mm Hg (ref. pg. 59)
8. 6 mm Hg (ref. pg. 60)
9. decrease (ref. pg. 61)
10. greater (ref. pg. 61)
11. below (ref. pg. 62)
12. 3 to 6, 2 to 4 (ref. pg. 62)

STATIC CHARACTERISTICS OF THE LUNGS

1. study of matter at rest and the forces bringing about or maintaining equilibrium (ref. pg. 62)
2. collapse (ref. pg. 62)
3. expand (ref. pgs. 62–63)
4. a. the elastic properties of the lung tissue
   b. surface tension produced by the layer of fluid that lines the inside of the alveoli (ref. pg. 63)

ELASTIC PROPERTIES OF THE LUNGS

1. volume, pressure (ref. pg. 63)

Case A

2. a. (ref. pg. 63)
      .055 L/cm H_2O (55 ml/cm H_2O)
   b. .070 L/cm H_2O (70 ml/cm H_2O)
   c. Increasing

Case B

3. a. (ref. pgs. 63)
   .050 L/cm H_2O (50 ml/cm H_2O)
   b. .045 L/cm H_2O (45 ml/cm H_2O)
   c. decreasing
4. 0.1 L/cm H_2O (ref. pg. 63)
5. 2000 ml (2 liters) (ref. pg. 64)
6. right (ref. pg. 65)
7. a (ref. pg. 65)
8. b (ref. pg. 64)
9. the natural ability of matter to respond directly to force and to return to its original resting position or shape after the external force no longer exists (ref. pgs, 63–65)
10. the change in pressure per change in volume

    Elastance $= \dfrac{\Delta P}{\Delta V}$ (ref. pg. 65)

11. low, high (ref. pg. 65)
12. when a truly elastic body, like a spring, is acted on by 1 unit of force, the elastic body will stretch 1 unit of length, and when acted on by 2 units of force it will stretch 2 units of length, and so forth (ref. pg. 65)
13. volume, pressure (ref. pg. 65)
14. surface tension (ref. pg. 68)
15. 70 dynes/cm (ref. pg. 68)

16. $P = \dfrac{2ST}{r}$ (ref. pg. 69)

17. a. directly proportional to the surface tension of the liquid
    b. inversely proportional to the radius of the sphere (ref. pg. 69)
18. increases, decreases (ref. pg. 69)
19. b (ref. pg. 69)
20. critical opening pressure (ref. pg. 70)
21. c (ref. pg. 72)
22. alveolar type II cells (ref. pg. 73)
23. water insoluble, water soluble (ref. pg. 73)
24. increases, decrease (ref. pg. 73)
25. 1–5 dynes, 50 dynes (ref. pg. 74)
26. a. acidosis
    b hypoxia
    c. hyperoxia
    d. atelectasis
    e. pulmonary vascular congestion (ref. pg. 76)
27. low (ref. pg. 76)

DYNAMIC CHARACTERISTICS OF THE LUNGS

1. study of forces in action (ref. pg. 78)
2. the movement of in action gas in and out of the lungs and the pressure changes required to move the gas (ref. pg. 78).

3. $\dot{V} \approx \dfrac{\Delta P r^4 \pi}{81 \eta}$ (ref. pg. 79)

4. a. increases
   b. increases
   c. increases
   d. increases (ref. pg. 79)
5. a. 2 liters/minute (L/min)
   b. 14 L/min
   c. 256 cm H_2O
   d. 20 cm H_2O
   e. 800 L/min
   f. 200 L/min
   g. 5 cm H_2O
   h. 2.5 cm H_2O (ref. pg. 79)

6. $\dot{V} \approx P r^4$

   $P \approx \dfrac{\dot{V}}{r^4}$ (ref. pg. 81)

AIRWAY RESISTANCE AND DYNAMIC COMPLIANCE

1. pressure difference between the mouth and the alveoli divided by flow rate (ref. pg. 82)

2. $R_{aw} = \dfrac{\Delta P(\text{cm } H_2O)}{\dot{V}(\text{L/sec})}$ (ref. pg. 82)

3. 3 cm H_2O/L/sec (ref. pg. 82)
4. 1.0, 2.0 (ref. pg. 83)
5. a gas flow that is streamlined (ref. pg. 83)
6. molecules that move through a tube in a random manner (ref. pg. 83)
7. time (in seconds) necessary to inflate a particular lung region to 60 percent of its potential filling capacity (ref. pg. 84)
8. b (ref. pg. 84)
9. b (ref. pg. 84)
10. c (ref. pg. 84)
11. a (ref. pg. 84)
12. a (ref. pg. 84)
13. e (ref. pg. 84)
14. change in the volume of the lungs divided by the change in the transpulmonary pressure during the time required for one breath (ref. pg. 84)

15. equal to (ref. pg. 85)
16. decreases (ref. pg. 86)
17. alveoli distal to an obstruction that do not have enough time to fill to their potential filling capacity as the breathing frequency increases (ref. pg. 86)

VENTILATORY PATTERNS

1. a. tidal volume
   b. ventilatory rate
   c. time relationship between inhalation and exhalation (ref. pg. 86)
2. 7 to 9, 3 to 4 (ref. pg. 86)
3. 15 (ref. pg. 86)
4. 1 : 2 (ref. pg. 86)
5. alveolar ventilation (ref. pg. 87)
6. deadspace ventilation (ref. pg. 87)
7. the volume of gas in the conducting airways: The nose, mouth, pharynx, larynx and lower airways down to, but not including, the respiratory bronchioles (ref. pg. 88)
8. 130 ml (ref. pg. 88)
9. tidal volume, deadspace ventilation, breaths per minute (ref. pg. 89)
10. 6240 ml (ref. pg. 89)
11. an alveolus that is ventilated but not perfused with pulmonary blood (ref. pg. 91)
12. the sum of the anatomic deadspace and alveolar deadspace (ref. pg. 91)
13. greater (ref. pg. 91)
14. greater (ref. pg. 91)
15. c (ref. pg. 91)
16. increases, decreases (ref. pg. 91)
17. decreases, increases (ref. pg. 92)
18. energy, ventilation (ref. pg. 93)
19. complete absence of spontaneous ventilation (ref. pg. 94)
20. normal, spontaneous breathing (ref. pg. 95)
21. short episodes of rapid, uniformly deep inspirations, followed by 10 to 30 seconds of apnea (ref. pg. 95)
22. increased depth of breathing with or without an increased frequency (ref. pg. 95)
23. an increased alveolar ventilation produced by any ventilatory pattern that causes the $P_{A_{CO_2}}$ and, therefore, the Pa_{CO_2} to decrease (ref. pg. 96)
24. a decreased alveolar ventilation produced by any ventilatory pattern that causes the $P_{A_{CO_2}}$ and, therefore, the Pa_{CO_2} to increase (ref. pg. 96)
25. a rapid breathing rate (ref. pg. 96)
26. 10 to 30 seconds of apnea, followed by a gradual increase in the volume and frequency of breathing, followed by a gradual decrease in the volume of breathing until another period of apnea occurs (ref. pg. 97)
27. both an increased depth and rate of breathing (ref. pg. 97)
28. a condition in which an individual is able to breathe most comfortably in the upright position (ref. pg. 98)
29. difficulty in breathing, of which the individual is consciously aware (ref. pg. 98)

CHAPTER THREE

THE DIFFUSION OF PULMONARY GASES

ANSWERS

DIFFUSION AND GAS LAWS

1. the movement of gas molecules from an area of relatively high concentration of gas to one of low concentration (ref. pg. 108)
2. if temperature remains constant, pressure will vary inversely to volume (ref. pg. 109)
3. $P_1 \times V_1 = P_2 \times V_2$ (ref. pg. 109)
4. 66.66 cm H_2O (ref. pg. 109)
5. 37.5 cm H_2O (ref. pg. 109)
6. if pressure remains constant, volume and temperature will vary directly (ref. pg. 109)
7. $V_1/T_1 = V_2/T_2$ (ref. pg. 109)
8. 9.37 L (ref. pg. 109)
9. 4.64 L (ref. pg. 109)
10. if the volume remains constant, pressure and temperature will vary directly (ref. pg. 109)
11. $P_1/T_1 = P_2/T_2$ (ref. pg. 109)
12. 156.2 cm H_2O (ref. pg. 109)
13. 44.53 cm H_2O (ref. pg. 109)
14. in a mixture of gases, the total pressure is equal to the sum of the partial pressures of each separate gas (ref. pg. 109)
15. 650 mm Hg (ref. pg. 109)

THE PARTIAL PRESSURES OF ATMOSPHERIC GASES

1. (ref. pg. 111)
2. decreases, remains the same (ref. pg. 110)
3. (ref. pg. 111)
4. the alveolar oxygen must mix—or compete in terms of partial pressures—with alveolar CO_2 pressure and alveolar water vapor pressure (ref. pg. 111)
5. 44 mg/L, 47 mm Hg (ref. pg. 112)
6. 428.2 mm Hg (ref. pg. 112)

THE DIFFUSION OF PULMONARY GASES

1. a. liquid lining the intra-alveolar membrane
   b. alveolar epithelial cell
   c. basement membrane of the alveolar epithelial cell
   d. loose connective tissue (the interstitial space)
   e. basement membrane of the capillary endothelium
   f. capillary endothelium
   g. plasma in the capillary blood
   h. erythrocyte membrane
   i. intracellular fluid in the erythrocyte (ref. pg. 113)
2. 0.36 to 2.5 μ (ref. pg. 114)
3. 40, 46 (ref. pg. 114)
4. 60, 6 (ref. pg. 114)
5. 0.25 (ref. pg. 116)
6. 0.75, one-third (ref. pg. 116)
7. b (ref. pg. 116)

8. $\dot{V}gas = \dfrac{AD(P_1 - P_2)}{T}$ (ref. pg. 118)

9. a. a
   b. a
   c. b (ref. pg. 118)
10. the amount of gas that dissolves in a liquid at a given temperature is proportional to the partial pressure of the gas (ref. pg. 118)
11. solubility coefficient (ref. pg. 118)
12. a. directly proportional to the solubility coefficient of the gas
    b. inversely proportional to the square root of the gram-molecular weight of the gas (ref. pg. 119)

PERFUSION- AND DIFFUSION-LIMITED GAS FLOW

1. the transfer of gas across the alveolar wall is a function of the amount of blood that flows past the alveoli (ref. pg. 120)
2. the movement of gas across the alveolar wall is a function of the integrity of the alveolar-capillary membrane itself (ref. pg. 120)
3. a (ref. pg. 124)

CHAPTER FOUR

PULMONARY FUNCTION MEASUREMENTS

ANSWERS

LUNG VOLUMES AND CAPACITIES

1. the volume of air that normally moves into and out of the lungs in one quiet breath (ref. pg. 130)
2. the maximum volume of air that can be inhaled after a normal tidal volume inhalation (ref. pg. 130)
3. the maximum volume of air that can be exhaled after a normal tidal volume exhalation (ref. pg. 130)
4. the amount of air remaining in the lungs after a maximal exhalation (ref. pg. 130)
5. the maximum volume of air that can be exhaled after a maximal inspiration (ref. pg. 131)
6. the volume of air that can be inhaled after a normal exhalation (ref. pg. 131)
7. the volume of air remaining in the lungs after a normal exhalation (ref. pg. 131)
8. maximum amount of air that the lungs can accommodate (ref. pg. 131)
9. the percentage of the TLC occupied by the RV (ref. pg. 131)
10. (ref. pg. 131)
11. RV, V_T, FRC, RV/TLC ratio; VC, IC, IRV, ERV (ref. pg. 133)
12. VC, IC, RV, FRC, V_T, TLC (ref. pg. 133)

PULMONARY MECHANICS

1. the maximum volume of gas that can be exhaled as forcefully and rapidly as possible after a maximal inspiration (ref. pg. 133)
2. the maximum volume of gas that can be exhaled over a specific period of time (ref. pg. 133)
3. a. 60%
   b. 83%
   c. 94%
   d. 97% (ref. pg. 134)
4. decreases (ref. pg. 134)
5. the average rate of airflow between 200 and 1200 ml of the FVC (ref. pg. 134)
6. large (ref. pg. 134)
7. the average flow rate during the middle 50% of an FVC measurement (ref. pg. 136)
8. medium, small (ref. pg. 136)

9. the maximum flow rate that can be achieved (ref. pg. 136)
10. the largest volume of gas that can be breathed voluntarily in and out of the lungs in 1 minute (ref. pg. 136)
11. the ratio of the volume of gas that can be forcefully exhaled in 1 second to the total volume of gas that can be forcefully exhaled after a maximum inspiration (ref. pg. 138)
12. (ref. pg. 139)
13. (ref. pg. 141)

EFFECTS OF DYNAMIC COMPRESSION ON EXPIRATORY FLOW RATES

1. the initial flow rate during forced expiration depends on the muscular effort produced by the individual (ref. pg. 141)
2. once a maximum flow rate has been attained, the flow rate cannot be increased by further muscular effort (ref. pg. 141)
3. dynamic compression (ref. pg. 141)
4. toward the alveolus (upstream) (ref. pg. 141)
5. increases (ref. pg. 141)

CHAPTER FIVE

THE CIRCULATORY SYSTEM

ANSWERS

BLOOD

1. a. plasma
   b. erythrocytes
   c. leukocytes
   d. thrombocytes (ref. pg. 152)
2. erythrocytes (ref. pg. 153)
3. 5 (ref. pg. 153)
4. 4 (ref. pg. 153)
5. hematocrit (ref. pg. 153)
6. a. 45%
   b. 42%
   c. 45 to 60% (ref. pgs. 154)
7. 7.5 μ, 2.5 μ (ref. pg. 154)
8. 120 (ref. pg. 154)
9. Protect the body against the invasion of bacteria and other foreign agents that can harm the body (ref. pg. 154)
10. 5000 to 9000 (ref. pg. 154)
11. (ref. pg. 154)
12. neutrophils (ref. pg. 154)
13. eosinophils (ref. pg. 154)
14. monocytes (ref. pg. 154)
15. lymphocytes (ref. pg. 155)
16. platelets (ref. pg. 155)
17. 250,000 and 500,000 (ref. pg. 155)
18. prevent blood loss from a traumatized surface of the body involving the smallest vessels (ref. pg. 155)
19. 55 (ref. pg. 155)
20. 90 (ref. pg. 155)
21. a. albumins
    b. Na^+
    b. K^+
    c. Ca^{2+}
    d. Mg^{2+} (ref. pg. 155)

23. a. Cl^-
    b. PO_4^{3-}
    c. SO_4^{2-}
    d. HCO_3^- (ref. pg. 155)
24. a. amino acids
    b. glucose/carbohydrates
    c. lipids
    d. individual vitamins (ref. pg. 155)
25. a. urea
    b. creatinine
    c. uric acid
    d. bilirubin (ref. pg. 155)

THE HEART

1. (ref. pg. 156)
2. inferior and superior vena cava (ref. pg. 157)
3. tricuspid valve (ref. pg. 157)
4. papillary muscles (ref. pg. 157)
5. pulmonary trunk, pulmonary arteries (ref. pg. 157)
6. pulmonary veins (ref. pg. 158)
7. mitral valve (ref. pg. 158)
8. aorta (ref. pg. 158)
9. aortic (ref. pg. 158)
10. (ref. pg. 159)
11. sinoatrial node (ref. pg. 158)
12. sympathetic (ref. pg. 159)
13. parasympathetic (ref. pg. 159)
14. depolarization of the atria (ref. pg. 160)
15. ventricular depolarization (ref. pg. 160)
16. ventricular repolarization (ref. pg. 160)
17. (ref. pg. 161)
18. 60–100 beats/min (ref. pg. 161)
19. 130–140 beats/min (ref. pg. 161)

THE PULMONARY AND SYSTEMIC VASCULAR SYSTEMS

1. pulmonary trunk, left atrium (ref. pg. 161)
2. aorta, right atrium (ref. pg. 161)
3. away from (ref. pg. 161)
4. arterioles (ref. pg. 161)
5. arterioles (ref. pg. 161)
6. arterioles (ref. pg. 161)
7. external (ref. pg. 161)
8. internal (ref. pg. 161)

9. venules (ref. pg. 161)
10. capacitance (ref. pg. 163)
11. 60 (ref. pg. 163)
12. sympathetic (ref. pg. 163)
13. vasomotor, medulla oblongata, sympathetic (ref. pg. 163)
14. sympathetic (ref. pg. 163)
15. vasomotor tone (ref. pg. 163)
16. increasing, sympathetic (ref. pg. 163)
17. decreasing, sympathetic (ref. pg. 163)
18. a. heart
    b. brain
    c. skeletal muscles (ref. pg. 163)
19. pressoreceptors (ref. pg. 164)
20. glossopharyngeal (ref. pg. 164)
21. vagus (ref. pg. 164)
22. decrease, increase (ref. pg. 164)
23. a. an increased cardiac output
    b. an increase in the total peripheral resistance
    c. the return of blood pressure toward normal (ref. pg. 164)
24. a. large arteries
    b. large veins
    c. pulmonary vessels
    d. cardiac walls (ref. pg. 164)

PRESSURES IN THE PULMONARY AND SYSTEMIC VASCULAR SYSTEMS

1. actual blood pressure in the lumen of any vessel at any point relative to the barometric pressure (ref. pg. 166)
2. difference between the pressure in the lumen of a vessel and the pressure surrounding the vessel (ref. pg. 166)
3. greater than (ref. pg. 166)
4. less than (ref. pg. 166)
5. pressure difference between the pressure at one point in a vessel and the pressure at any other point downstream in the vessel (ref. pg. 166)

THE CARDIAC CYCLE AND ITS EFFECT ON BLOOD PRESSURE

1. systolic pressure (ref. pg. 167)
2. diastolic pressure (ref. pg. 167)
3. 10 (ref. pg. 167)
4. (ref. pg. 169)
5. 40 ml and 80 ml (ref. pg. 168)

6. cardiac output (ref. pg. 168)
7. 4400 ml (ref. pg. 169)
8. a (ref. pg. 169)
9. 5 (ref. pg. 169)
10. 75, 15, 10 (ref. pg. 169)
11. 60, 10 (ref. pgs. 169–70)

THE DISTRIBUTION OF PULMONARY BLOOD FLOW

1. to the portion of the body, or portion of the organ, that is closest to the ground (ref. pg. 170)
2. greater than (ref. pg. 171)
3. a. posterior
   b. anterior
   c. lung nearest the ground
   d. apices (ref. pg. 172)
4. greater than (ref. pg. 171)
5. a. severe hemorrhage
   b. dehydration
   c. positive pressure ventilation (ref. pg. 172)
6. alveolar dead space (ref. pg. 172)
7. greater than, greater than (ref. pg. 172)
8. greater than, less than (ref. pg. 173)
9. a. ventricular preload
   b. ventricular afterload
   c. myocardial contractility (ref. pg. 174)
10. the degree to which the myocardial fiber is stretched prior to contraction (ref. pg. 174)
11. more (ref. pg. 174)
12. ventricular end-diastolic pressure (ref. pg. 174)
13. ventricular end-diastolic volume (ref. pg. 174)
14. a (ref. pg. 174)
15. Frank-Starling relationship (ref. pg. 174)
16. the force against which the ventricles must work to pump blood (ref. pg. 174)
17. a. the volume and viscosity of blood ejected
    b. peripheral vascular resistance
    c. total cross-sectional area of the vascular space into which blood is ejected (ref. pg. 174)
18. arterial systolic blood pressure (ref. pg. 174)

19. $BP = CO \times SVR$ (ref. pg. 174)

20. the force generated by the myocardium when the ventricular muscle fibers shorten (ref. pg. 174)
21. b (ref. pg. 174)
22. a. pulse
    b. blood pressure
    c. skin temperature
    d. serial hemodynamic measurements (ref. pg. 174)
23. positive inotropism (ref. pg. 174)
24. negative inotropism (ref. pg. 174)

25. $\text{resistance} = \dfrac{\text{mean blood pressure}}{\text{cardiac output}}$ (ref. pg. 175)

26. a (ref. pg. 175)

ACTIVE MECHANISMS AFFECTING VASCULAR RESISTANCE

1. the physiologic, pharmacologic, or pathologic processes that have a direct effect on the vascular system (ref. pg. 176)
2. a (ref. pg. 176)
3. a (ref. pg. 176)
4. a (ref. pg. 176)
5. a (ref. pg. 176)
6. a. epinephrine (Adrenalin)
   b. norepinephrine (Levophed)
   c. dobutamine (Dobutrex)
   d. dopamine (Intropin)
   e. phenylephrine (Neo-Synephrine) (ref. pg. 176)
7. a. oxygen
   b. isoproterenol (Isuprel)
   c. aminophylline
   d. calcium-blocking agents (ref. pg. 176)
8. a. vessel blockage or obstruction
   b. vessel wall diseases
   c. vessel destruction or obliteration
   d. vessel compression (ref. pg. 177)

PASSIVE MECHANISMS AFFECTING VASCULAR RESISTANCE

1. a secondary change in pulmonary vascular resistance that occurs in response to another mechanical change (ref. pg. 177)
2. b (ref. pg. 177)
3. the opening of vessels that were closed, the stretching or widening of vessels that were open (ref. pg. 177)
4. b (ref. pg. 177)
5. high (ref. pg. 179)
6. low (ref. pg. 179)
7. low (ref. pg. 179)
8. high (ref. pg. 179)
9. low (ref. pg. 179)
10. high (ref. pg. 179)
11. b (ref. pg. 181)
12. a (ref. pg. 181)

CHAPTER SIX

HEMODYNAMIC MEASUREMENTS

ANSWERS

HEMODYNAMIC MEASUREMENTS DIRECTLY OBTAINED BY MEANS OF THE PULMONARY ARTERY CATHETER

1. the study of the forces that influence the circulation of blood (ref. pg. 189)
2. (ref. pg. 191)

HEMODYNAMIC VALUES COMPUTED FROM DIRECT MEASUREMENTS

1. (ref. pg. 191)
2. the volume of blood ejected by the ventricles with each contraction (ref. pg. 199)
3. a. preload
   b. afterload
   c. myocardial contractility (ref. pg. 191)

4. $SV = \dfrac{CO}{HR}$ (ref. pg. 192)

5. 63.21 ml/beat (ref. pg. 192)
6. dividing the stroke volume (SV) by the body surface area (BSA) (ref. pg. 193)
7. 22 ml/beat/m² (ref. pg. 193)
8. a. contractility of the heart
   b. overall blood volume status
   c. degree of venous return (ref. pg. 193)
9. dividing the cardiac output (CO) by the body's surface area (BSA) (ref. pg. 193)
10. 2.8 L/min/m² (ref. pg. 193)
11. the amount of work required by the right ventricle to pump blood (ref. pg. 193)
12. contractility of the right ventricle (ref. pg. 193)

13. $RVSWI = SVI \times (\overline{PA} - CVP) \times 0.0136 \text{ g/ml}$ (ref. pg. 194)

14. 8.16 g m/m² (ref. pg. 194)
15. the amount of work required by the left ventricle to pump blood (ref. pg. 194)
16. contractility of the left ventricle (ref. pg. 194)

17. LVSWI = SVI × (MAP − PCWP) × 0.0136 g/ml   (ref. pg. 194)

18. 70.38 g m/m² (ref. pg. 194)
19. (ref. pg. 194)
20. low (ref. pg. 194)
21. high (ref. pg. 194)
22. the afterload of the right ventricle (ref. pg. 195)

23. PVR = $\dfrac{\overline{PA} - PCWP \times 80}{CO}$ (ref. pg. 195)

24. 114 dynes × sec cm⁻⁵ (ref. pg. 195)
25. (ref. pg. 196)
26. (ref. pg. 196)
27. the afterload of the left ventricle (ref. pg. 195)

28. SVR = $\dfrac{MAP - CVP \times 80}{CO}$ (ref. pg. 196)

29. 1266 dynes × sec cm⁻⁵ (ref. pg. 195)
30. (ref. pg. 197)

CHAPTER SEVEN

OXYGEN TRANSPORT

ANSWERS

OXYGEN TRANSPORT

1. (ref. pg. 205)

Blood Gas Value	Arterial	Venous
pH	7.35–7.45	7.30–7.40
P_{CO_2}	35–45 mm Hg	42–48 mm Hg
HCO_3^-	22–28 mEq/L	24–30 mEq/L
P_{O_2}	80–100 mm Hg	35–45 mm Hg

2. maintains its precise molecular structure and freely moves throughout the plasma in its normal gaseous state (ref. pg. 204)
3. dissolved O_2 (ref. pg. 204)
4. a. 0.15
   b. 0.15 vol% (ref. pg. 205)
5. the amount of O_2 in ml that is in 100 ml of blood (ref. pg. 205)
6. 280 (ref. pg. 205)
7. A (ref. pg. 205)
8. four (ref. pg. 205)

9. $Hb + O_2 \rightleftharpoons Hb_{O_2}$ (ref. pg. 205)

10. 50, 25 (ref. pg. 206)
11. oxyhemoglobin (ref. pg. 206)
12. reduced hemoglobin or deoxyhemoglobin (ref. pg. 206)
13. directly (ref. pg. 206)
14. two identical α chains, each with 141 amino acids, and two identical β chains, each with 146 amino acids ($\alpha_2\beta_2$) (ref. pg. 206)
15. two α, two γ (ref. pg. 206)
16. methemoglobin (ref. pg. 206)
17. a. 14–16
    b. 12–15
    c. 14–20 (ref. pg. 206)

18. 33 (ref. pg. 207)
19. 1.34 (ref. pg. 207)
20. a Thebesian venous drainage into the left atrium
    b. bronchial venous drainage into the pulmonary veins
    c. alveoli that are underventilated in proportion to pulmonary blood flow (ref. pg. 207)
21. **Case A**
    a. 0.165
    b. 14.807
    c. 14.972
    d. 149.72
    e. 898.32 (ref. pg. 207)
    Case B
    a. 0.15
    b. 19.296
    c. 19.446
    d. 194.46
    e. 680.61
    f. 12.135
    g. 24.57 (ref. pg. 207)

OXYGEN DISSOCIATION CURVE

1. percentage, pressure (ref. pg. 208)
2. a. the hemoglobin has an excellent safety zone for the loading of oxygen in the lungs
   b. the diffusion of oxygen during the transit time hemoglobin is in the alveolar-capillary system is enhanced
   c. increasing the P_{O_2} beyond 100 mm Hg adds very little additional oxygen to the blood (ref. pg. 209)
3. a. P_{O_2} reductions below 60 mm Hg indicate a rapid decrease in the amount of oxygen bound to hemoglobin
   b. a large amount of oxygen is released from the hemoglobin for only a small decrease in P_{O_2} (ref. pg. 210)
4. a 85%
   b. 17 vol% (ref. pg. 209)
5. the partial pressure at which the hemoglobin is 50% saturated with oxygen (ref. pg. 210)
6. 27 (ref. pg. 210)
7. a (ref. pg. 210)
8. b (ref. pg. 210)
9. a. ↑ pH
      ↓ P_{CO_2}
      ↓ temperature
      ↓ DPG
      HbF
      CO_{Hb} (ref. pgs. 210–13)

b. ↓ pH
$\uparrow P_{CO_2}$
↑ temperature
↑ DPG (ref. pgs. 210–13)
10. b (ref. pg. 214)
11. a (ref. pg. 216)
12. a (ref. pg. 217)
13. b (ref. pg. 218)

OXYGEN TRANSPORT STUDIES

1. a. total oxygen delivery
   b. arterial-venous oxygen content difference
   c. oxygen consumption
   d. oxygen extraction ratio
   e. mixed venous oxygen saturation
   f. pulmonary shunting (ref. pg. 220)
2. a. body's ability to oxygenate blood
   b. hemoglobin concentration
   c. cardiac output (ref. pg. 220)

3. $D_{O_2} = Q_T \times (Ca_{O_2} \times 10)$ (ref. pg. 220)

4. 420 ml O_2/min (ref. pg. 220)
5. a. decline in blood oxygenation
   b. decline in hemoglobin concentration
   c. decline in cardiac output (ref. pg. 220)
6. between the Ca_{O_2} and the $C\bar{v}_{O_2}$ (ref. pg. 220)

7. $C(a - \bar{v})_{O_2} = Ca_{O_2} - C\bar{v}_{O_2}$ (ref. pg. 220)

8. 4 vol% (ref. pg. 220)
9. a. decreased cardiac output
   b. periods of increased oxygen consumption
      1. exercise
      2. seizures
      3. shivering post-operative patient
      4. hyperthermia (ref. pg. 222)
10. a. increased cardiac output
    b. skeletal relaxation
    c. peripheral shunting
    d. certain poisons (cyanide)
    e. hypothermia (ref. pg. 222)
11. oxygen consumption, oxygen uptake (ref. pg. 221)

12. $\dot{V}_{O_2} = QT[C(a - \bar{v})_{O_2} \times 10]$ (ref. pg. 222)

13. 600 ml O_2/min (ref. pg. 222)

14. a. exercise
    b. seizures
    c. shivering in postoperative patient
    d. hyperthermia (ref. pg. 223)
15. a. skeletal relaxation
    b. peripheral shunting
    c. certain poisons (cyanide)
    d. hypothermia (ref. pg. 223)
16. body surface area (BSA) (ref. pg. 222)
17. 125, 165 (ref. pg. 222)
18. extracted by the peripheral tissues divided by the amount of oxygen delivered to the peripheral cells (ref. pg. 222)
19. a. oxygen coefficient ratio
    b. oxygen utilization ratio (ref. pg. 223)

20. $O_2ER = \dfrac{Ca_{O_2} - C\bar{v}_{O_2}}{CaO_2}$ (ref. pg. 223)

21. 25 (ref. pg. 233)
22. a. 50 (ref. pg. 223)
    b. 425, 425 (ref. pg. 223)
23. a. decreased cardiac output
    b. period of increased oxygen consumption
       1. exercise
       2. seizures
       3. shivering in postoperative patient
       4. hyperthermia
    c. anemia
    d. decreased arterial oxygenation (ref. pg. 224)
24. a. increased cardiac output
    b. peripheral shunting
    c. certain poisons (cyanide)
    d. hypothermia
    e. increased hemoglobin concentration
    f. increased arterial oxygenation (ref. pg. 224)
25. 75 (ref. pg. 224)
26. 65 (ref. pg. 224)
27. a. decreased cardiac output
    b. periods of increased oxygen consumption
       1. exercises
       2. seizures
       3. shivering in postoperative patient
       4. hyperthermia (ref. pg. 225)
28. a (ref. pg. 225)
29. a. increased cardiac output
    b. skeletal relaxation
    c. peripheral shunting
    d. certain poisons (cyanide)
    e. hypothermia (ref. pg. 225)

30. b (ref. pg. 225)
31. (ref. pg. 226)

MECHANISMS OF PULMONARY SHUNTING

1. that portion of the cardiac output that enters the left side of the heart without exchanging gases with the alveolar gases—or the blood that does exchange gases with alveolar gases but does not obtain a P_{O_2} that equals the alveolus (ref. pg. 225)
2. a. anatomic shunts
   b. capillary shunts (ref. pg. 225)
3. blood flows from the right side of the heart to the left side without coming in contact with an alveolus for gas exchange (ref. pg. 225)
4. 2, 5 (ref. pg. 225)
5. a. congenital heart disease
   b. intrapulmonary fistula
   c. vascular lung tumors (ref. pg. 226)
6. a. alveolar collapse or atelectasis
   b. alveolar fluid accumulation
   c. alveolar consolidation (ref. pg. 226)
7. true, absolute shunt (ref. pg. 226)
8. the hypoxemia produced by an absolute shunt cannot be treated by simply increasing the concentration of inspired oxygen, since the alveoli are unable to accommodate any form of ventilation (ref. pg. 226)
9. pulmonary capillary perfusion is in excess of alveolar ventilation (ref. pg. 228)
10. a. hypoventilation
    b. uneven distribution of ventilation
    c. alveolar-capillary diffusion defects (ref. pg. 228)
11. the mixing of shunted, non-reoxygenated blood with reoxygenated blood distal to the alveoli (ref. pg. 228)
12. $\dfrac{\dot{Q}s}{\dot{Q}T} = \dfrac{Cc_{O_2} - Ca_{O_2}}{Cc_{O_2} - C\bar{v}_{O_2}}$ (ref. pg. 229)
13. a. 268.1 mm Hg
    b. 14.204 vol% $_{O_2}$
    c. 12.389 vol% $_{O_2}$
    d. 8.139 vol% $_{O_2}$
    e. .29 (ref. pg. 229)
14. a. reflects normal lung status
    b. reflects an intrapulmonary abnormality
    c. reflects significant intrapulmonary disease, and may be life-threatening in patients with limited cardiovascular or central nervous system function
    d. reflects a potentially life-threatening situation—aggressive cardiopulmonary support is generally required (ref. pg. 230)
15. a. questionable perfusion status
    b. decreased myocardial reserve
    c. unstable oxygen consumption demand (ref. pg. 231)

TISSUE HYPOXIA

1. the condition in which the Pa_{O_2} and Ca_{O_2} are abnormally low (ref. pg. 231)
2. a. low alveolar P_{O_2}
   b. diffusion impairment
   c. ventilation/perfusion mismatch (ref. pg. 231)
3. a condition in which the oxygen tension in the arterial blood is normal, but the oxygen-carrying capacity of the blood is inadequate (ref. pg. 232)
4. a. low amount of hemoglobin in the blood
   b. deficiency in the ability for hemoglobin to carry oxygen (ref. pg. 232)
5. a condition in which the arterial blood that reaches the tissue cells may have a normal oxygen tension and content, but the blood is not adequate to meet tissue needs (ref. pg. 232)
6. a. stagnant hypoxia
   b. arterial-venous shunting (ref. pg. 232)
7. any condition that impairs the ability of tissue cells to utilize oxygen (ref. pg. 232)
8. the term used to describe the blue-gray or purplish discoloration seen on the mucous membranes, fingertips, and toes (ref. pg. 233)
9. an increased level of red blood cells (ref. pg. 234)

CHAPTER EIGHT

CARBON DIOXIDE TRANSPORT AND ACID BASE BALANCE

ANSWERS

CARBON DIOXIDE TRANSPORT

1. a. carbamino compound
   b. bicarbonate
   c. dissolved CO_2 (ref. pg. 242)
2. a. dissolved CO_2
   b. carbamino-Hb
   c. bicarbonate (ref. pg. 243)
3. bicarbonate (ref. pg. 244)
4. 63 (ref. pg. 244)
5. (ref. pg. 243)
6. linear (ref. pg. 246)

CARBON DIOXIDE ELIMINATION AT THE LUNGS

1. 40, 50 (ref. pg. 247)

CARBON DIOXIDE DISSOCIATION CURVE AND ACID-BASE BALANCE

1. Haldane effect (ref. pg. 246)
2. charged species (ions) that can conduct a current in solution (ref. pg. 249)
3. substance that is capable of neutralizing both acids and bases without causing an appreciable change in the original pH (ref. pg. 249)
4. dissociates completely into H^+ and an anion (ref. pg. 249)
5. dissociates only partially into ions (ref. pg. 249)
6. dissociates completely (ref. pg. 249)
7. reacts with water to form OH^- in an equilibrium; partial dissociation (ref. pg. 249)

8. weak acid or base systems that have an equilibrium between the molecular form and its ions (ref. pg. 249)
9. $[H^+] + [A^-]$ (ref. pg. 249)
10. neutral (ref. pg. 249)
11. acidic (ref. pg. 249)
12. basic (ref. pg. 249)
13. the negative logarithm, to the base 10, of the hydrogen ion concentration (ref. pg. 249)

14. $pH = -\log_{10}[H^+]$ (ref. pg. 249)

15. 10^{-7} (ref. pg. 249)
16. donates (ref. pg. 249)
17. decreases (ref. pg. 249)
18. accepts (ref. pg. 249)
19. increases (ref. pg. 249)
20. a. the buffer systems of the blood and tissue
    b. the respiratory ability to regulate the elimination of CO_2
    c. the renal ability to regulate the excretion of hydrogen and reabsorption of bicarbonate ions (ref. pg. 249)
21. carbonic acid/sodium bicarbonate (ref. pg. 250)

22. $pK + \log \dfrac{[HCO_3^-]}{[H_2CO_3]}$ (ref. pg. 250)

23. the dissociation constant of the acid portion of the buffer combination (ref. pg. 250)
24. 6.1 (ref. pg. 250)
25. 20, 1 (ref. pg. 251)
26. b (ref. pg. 251)
27. c (ref. pg. 251)

THE ROLE OF THE P_{CO_2}/HCO_3^- pH RELATIONSHIP IN ACID-BASE BALANCE

1. a. increases
   b increases
   c. increases
   d. decreases
   e. decreases (ref. pg. 252)
2. d (ref. pg. 252)
3. a (ref. pg. 252)
4. a. decreases
   b. decreases
   c. decreases
   d. increases
   e. increases (ref. pg. 253)
5. a (ref. pg. 253)
6. b (ref. pg. 253)
7. false (ref. pg. 255)

8. b (ref. pg. 256)
9. a. lactic acidosis
   b. ketoacidosis
   c. renal failure (ref. pg. 257)
10. a (ref. pg. 257)
11. a (ref. pg. 257)
12. a. hypokalemia
    b. hypochloremia
    c. gastric suction or vomiting
    d. excessive administration of steroids
    e. excessive administration of sodium bicarbonate (ref. pg. 257)
13. (ref. pg. 253)
    a. 7.23, 29
    b. 7.58, 17 or 18
    c. a combination of both
       a base deficit
       12–14 mEq/L
    d. respiratory
       a base excess
       3–4 mEq/L

CHAPTER NINE

VENTILATION-PERFUSION RELATIONSHIPS

ANSWERS

VENTILATION-PERFUSION RATIO

1. 4 (ref. pg. 265)
2. 5 (ref. pg. 265)
3. 4 : 5, 0.8 (ref. pg. 265)
4. higher (ref. pg. 266)
5. lower (ref. pg. 266)
6. decreases (ref. pg. 266)
7. a. the amount of oxygen ventilated into the alveoli
   b. the amount of oxygen removal by capillary blood flow (ref. pg. 266)
8. a. the amount of carbon dioxide that diffuses into the alveoli from the capillary blood
   b. the amount of carbon dioxide removal out of the alveoli by means of ventilation (ref. pg. 266)
9. it washes out of the alveoli faster than it is replaced by the venous blood (ref. pg. 267)
10. it does not diffuse into the blood as fast as it enters the alveolus.
    The $P_{A_{O_2}}$ also increases because of the reduced $P_{A_{CO_2}}$ (ref. pg. 267)
11. a (ref. pg. 267)
12. oxygen moves out of the alveolus and into the pulmonary capillary blood faster than it is replenished by ventilation (ref. pg. 268)
13. it moves out of the capillary blood and into the alveolus faster than it is washed out of the alveolus (ref. pg. 268)
14. c (ref. pg. 268)
15. decreases (ref. pg. 270)
16. increases (ref. pg. 270)
17. decreases (ref. pg. 271)
18. gas exchange between the systemic capillaries and the tissue cells (ref. pg. 272)
19. 250 (ref. pg. 272)
20. 200 (ref. pg. 272)
21. ratio between the volume of oxygen consumed and the volume of carbon dioxide produced (ref. pg. 273)

22. $RQ = \dfrac{\dot{V}_{CO_2}}{\dot{V}_{O_2}}$ (ref. pg. 273)

23. gas exchange between the pulmonary capillaries and the alveoli (ref. pg. 273)
24. quantity of oxygen and carbon dioxide exchanged during a period of 1 minute (ref. pg. 273)
25. a. pulmonary emboli
    b. partial or complete obstruction in the pulmonary artery or arterioles
    c. extrinsic pressure on the pulmonary vessels
    d. destruction of the pulmonary vessels
    e. decreased cardiac output (ref. pg. 273)
26. a. obstructive lung disorder
    b. restrictive lung disorders
    c. hypoventilation from any cause (ref. pg. 273)

CHAPTER TEN

CONTROL OF VENTILATION

ANSWERS

THE RESPIRATORY COMPONENTS OF THE MEDULLA

1. a. Dorsal Respiratory Group
   b. Ventral Respiratory Group (ref. pg. 280)
2. a (ref. pg. 280)
3. c (ref. pg. 281)
4. b. VRG (ref. pg. 281)
5. the middle and lower pons (ref. pg. 281)
6. b (ref. pg. 281)
7. b (ref. pg. 281)

MONITORING SYSTEMS THAT INFLUENCE THE RESPIRATORY COMPONENTS OF THE MEDULLA

1. hydrogen ions [H+] (ref. pg. 282)
2. bilaterally and ventrally in the substance of the medulla (ref. pg. 282)
3. CO_2, H+, HCO_3^- (ref. pg. 282)

4. $CO_2 + H_2O \rightleftarrows H_2CO_3 \rightleftarrows H^+ + HCO_3^-$ (ref. pg. 282)

5. The central chemoreceptors transmit signals to the respiratory component in the medulla, which, in turn, increases alveolar ventilation (ref. pg. 282)
6. indirect, pH level of the CSF (ref. pg. 283)
7. special oxygen-sensitive cells that react to reductions of oxygen levels in the arterial blood (ref. pg. 283)
8. high in neck, at the bifurcation of the internal and external carotid arteries and on the aortic arch (ref. pg. 283)
9. glossopharyngeal (9th); vagus (10th) (ref. pg. 284)
10. a (ref. pg. 284)
11. 60 mm Hg (ref. pg.284)
12. 30 mm Hg (ref. pg. 284)
13. A chronically high CO_2 concentration in the CSF inactivates the H+ sensitivity of the central chemoreceptors. HCO_3^- moves into the CSF via the active transport mechanism and combines with H+, thus returning the pH to normal (ref. pg. 285)

14. a (ref. pg. 285)
15. a. chronic anemia
    b. carbon monoxide poisoning
    c. methemoglobinemia (ref. pg. 287)
16. a. decreased pH ($\uparrow$ H+ level)
    b. hypoperfusion
    c. increased temperature
    d. nicotine
    e. the direct effect of Pa_{CO_2} (ref. pg. 287)
24. a. peripheral vasoconstriction
    b. increased pulmonary vascular resistance
    c. systemic arterial hypertension
    d. tachycardia
    e. increase in left ventricular performance (ref. pg. 288)

REFLEXES THAT INFLUENCE VENTILATION

1. lung overinflation (ref. pg. 288)
2. inspiration to cease (ref. pg. 288)
3. lung compression or deflation (ref. pg. 288)
4. an increased rate of breathing (ref. pg. 288)
5. lung compression, or lung exposure to noxious gases (ref. pg. 289)
6. in the trachea, bronchi, and bronchioles (ref. pg. 289)
7. the ventilatory rate to increase (ref. pg. 289)
8. in the interstitial tissues between the pulmonary capillaries and the alveoli (ref. pg. 289)
9. a. pulmonary capillary congestion
   b. capillary hypertension
   c. edema of the alveolar walls
   d. humoral agents (serotonin)
   e. lung deflation
   f. emboli (ref. pg. 289)
10. rapid, shallow breathing (ref. pg. 289)
11. a decreased heart and ventilatory rate (ref. pg. 289)
12. an increased heart and ventilatory rate (ref. pg. 289)
13. a. may cause respirations to temporarily cease
    b. may cause a temporary cessation of breathing
    c. can cause an immediate cessation of breathing, followed by an episode of coughing
    d triggers an increased respiratory rate
    e. may increase ventilation (ref. pg. 289)

CHAPTER ELEVEN

CARDIOPULMONARY PHYSIOLOGY OF THE FETUS AND THE NEWBORN

ANSWERS

FETAL LUNG DEVELOPMENT

1. a. embryonic
   b. pseudoglandular
   c. canalicular
   d. terminal sac (ref. pg. 296)
2. 24th (ref. pg. 296)
3. 20 (ref. pg. 298)
4. 28th (ref. pg. 298)

PLACENTA

1. cotyledons (ref. pg. 298)
2. (ref. pg. 300)
3. umbilical arteries (ref. pg. 298)
4. 20, 55 (ref. pg. 299)
5. the decreased maternal P_{CO_2} is caused by the alveolar hyperventilation that develops as the growing infant restricts the mother's diaphragmatic excursion (ref. pg. 299)
6. a. maternal-fetal P_{O_2} gradient
   b. higher hemoglobin concentration in the fetal blood
   c. greater affinity of fetal hemoglobin for oxygen (ref. pg. 300)
7. 30, 40 (ref. pg. 301)
8. umbilical vein (ref. pg. 301)
9. a. the placenta itself is an actively metabolizing organ
   b. the permeability of the placenta varies from region to region with respect to respiratory gases
   c. the fetal and maternal vascular shunts (ref. pg. 301)

FETAL CIRCULATION

1. ductus venosus (ref. pg. 301)
2. foramen ovale (ref. pg. 301)
3. left ventricle, heart, brain (ref. pg. 301)
4. ductus arteriosus, aorta (ref. pg. 301)
5. 15, pulmonary veins (ref. pg. 301)
6. 20 (ref. pg. 301)

Matching
7. e
   c
   a
   b
   d (ref. pg. 301)
8. a. the placenta is passed by the mother
   b. the umbilical arteries atrophy and become the lateral umbilical ligaments
   c. the umbilical vein becomes the round ligament (ligamentum teres) of the liver
   d. the ductus venosus becomes the lagamentum venosum, which is a fibrous cord in the liver
   e. the flap on the foramen ovale usually closes and becomes a depression in the interatrial septum called the fossa ovalis
   f. the ductus arteriosus atrophies and becomes the ligamentum arteriosum (ref. pg. 301)
9. a. about one-third of the fluid is squeezed out of the lungs as the infant passes through the birth canal
   b. about one-third of the fluid is absorbed by the pulmonary capillaries
   c. about one-third of the fluid is removed by the lymphatic system (ref. pg. 303)
10. 24 (ref. pg. 303)
11. 12 (ref. pg. 303)

BIRTH

1. a. thermal
   b. tactile
   c. visual (ref. pg. 303)
2. −40 (ref. pg. 304)
3. 40 (ref. pg. 304)
4. .005 L/cm H_2O (ref. pg.304)
5. 30 cm H_2O/L/sec (ref. pg. 304)
6. a. the sudden increase in the alveolar P_{O_2}, which offsets the hypoxic vasoconstriction
   b. the mechanical increase in lung volume, which widens the caliber of the extra-alveolar vessels (ref. pg. 305)
7. As the pulmonary vascular resistance decreases, a greater amount of blood flows through the lungs, and therefore more blood returns to the left atrium. This causes the pressure in the left atrium to increase and the flap of the foramen ovale to close. (ref. pg. 305)
8. 45, 50 (ref. pg. 305)

9. When the ductus arteriosus remains open (permitting blood to pass through it), and the pulmonary vascular resistance is elevated, persistent pulmonary hypertension of the neonate is said to exist (ref. pg. 305)
10. persistent fetal circulation
11. a. bradykinin
    b. serotonin
    c. prostaglandin inhibitors (ref. pg. 305)

CONTROL OF VENTILATION IN THE NEWBORN

1. peripheral, central (ref. pg. 305)
2. decrease (ref. pg. 306)
3. respiratory slowing or apnea (ref. pg. 306)
4. marked hyperventilation (ref. pg. 306)
5. a deep inspiration that is elicited by lung inflation (ref. pg. 306)

INFORMAL CLINICAL PARAMETERS IN THE NEWBORN

1. (ref. pg. 307)
2. (ref. pg. 307)

CHAPTER TWELVE

RENAL FAILURE AND ITS EFFECTS ON THE CARDIOPULMONARY SYSTEM

ANSWERS

THE KIDNEYS

1. (ref. pg. 316)
2. (ref. pg. 317)
3. (ref. pg. 318)

URINE FORMATION

1. (ref. pg. 319)
2. a. proximal convoluted tubule
   b. loop of Henle
   c. distal convoluted tubule (ref. pg. 320)
3. proximal convoluted tubule (ref. pg. 320)
4. various substances are transported from the plasma of the peritubular capillaries to the fluid of the renal tubule (ref. pg. 320)
5. hydrogen (H^+), potassium (K^+) (ref. pg. 320)

URINE CONCENTRATION AND VOLUME

1. a. countercurrent mechanism
   b. selective permeability of the collecting duct (ref. pg. 320)
2. renal medulla (ref. pg. 320)
3. 300 (ref. pg. 320)
4. 300, 1200 (ref. pgs. 320–21)
5. hypothalamus, pituitary gland (ref. pgs. 321–22)
6. b (ref. pg. 322)
7. a (ref. pg. 322)

8. increases (ref. pg. 322)
9. decreases (ref. pg. 322)
10. 1.018 to 1.040 (ref. pg. 322)

REGULATION OF ELECTROLYTE CONCENTRATION

1. a. sodium
   b. potassium
   c. calcium, magnesium, and phosphate (ref. pg. 322)
2. hydrogen (ref. pg. 323)
3. sodium bicarbonate (ref. pg. 323)
4. a. capillary fluid shift system
   b. the renal system (ref. pg. 323)

RENAL FAILURE

1. a. unilateral renal agenesis
   b. renal dysplasia
   c. polycystic disease of the kidney (ref. pg. 325)
2. women (ref. pg. 325)
3. a. calculi
   b. normal pregnancy
   c. prostatic hypertrophy
   d. infection and inflammation causing scar tissue
   e. neurologic disorders (ref. pg. 325)
4. a. altered immune responses
   b. drugs and related chemicals
   c radiation (ref. pg. 326)
5. Wilms' tumor (ref. pg. 326)
6. a. hypovolemia
   b. septicemia
   c. heart failure
   d. renal artery atherosclerosis (ref. pg. 326)
7. a sharp reduction in urine output (ref. pg. 326)
8. a renal ischemia
   b. injury to the glomerular membrane caused by nephrotoxic agents
   c. acute tubular necrosis
   d. intratubular obstruction
   e. acute inflammatory conditions (ref. pg. 327)
9. a. ureteral obstruction (ref. pg. 327)
   b. bladder outlet obstruction
10. decreases (ref. pg. 327)
11. increases (ref. pg. 327)
12. a (ref. pg. 327)
13. b (ref. pg. 327)

CARDIOPULMONARY PROBLEMS CAUSED BY RENAL FAILURE

1. sodium (ref. pg. 328)
2. a. increases
   b. increases
   c. decreases (ref. pg. 328)
3. b (ref. pg. 328)
4. b (ref. pg. 328)
5. a (ref. pg. 328)
6. a (ref. pgs. 328–29)
7. a. the production of erythropoietin is often inadequate to stimulate the production of red blood cells
   b. toxic waste accumulation suppresses the ability of bone marrow to produce red blood cells (ref. pg. 329)
8. because of the platelet abnormalities associated with renal failure (ref. pg. 329)
9. this condition develops as a result of the pericardium exposure to the metabolic end-products associated with renal decline (ref. pg. 329)

CHAPTER THIRTEEN

AGING AND ITS EFFECTS ON THE CARDIOPULMONARY SYSTEM

ANSWERS

THE INFLUENCE OF AGING ON THE RESPIRATORY SYSTEM

1. 20 (ref. pg. 337)
2. 20, 25 (ref. pg. 337)
3. decreases, increases (ref. pg. 338)
4. a. increases
   b. decreases
   c. decreases
   d. remains the same
   e. increases
   f. increases
   g. decreases (ref. pg. 339)
5. a. decreases
   b. decreases
   c. decreases
   d. decreases
   e. decreases
   f. decreases (ref. pg. 340)
6. a. decreases (ref. pg. 340)
   b. increases (ref. pg. 340)
   c. increases (ref. pg. 340)
   d. decreases (ref. pg. 341)
   e. remains the same (ref. pg. 341)
   f. remains the same (ref. pg. 341)
   g. remains the same (ref. pg. 341)
   h. decreases (ref. pg. 341)
   i. decreases (ref. pg. 341)

ARTERIAL BLOOD GASES

1. b (ref. pg. 341)
2. b (ref. pg. 341)

THE INFLUENCE OF AGING ON THE CARDIOVASCULAR SYSTEM

1. b (ref. pg. 342)
2. b (ref. pg. 342)
3. b (ref. pg. 342)
4. 150 (ref. pg. 342)
5. a. decreases (ref. pg. 343)
   b. decreases (ref. pg. 343)
   c. increases (ref. pg. 344)
   d. increases (ref. pg. 344)
   e. increases (ref. pg. 344)

CHAPTER FOURTEEN

EXERCISE AND ITS EFFECTS ON THE CARDIOPULMONARY SYSTEM

ANSWERS

EFFECTS OF EXERCISE

1. a. 20
   b. 3
   c. 6
   d. 25
   e. 20
   f. 20 (ref. pg. 349)
2. 30, 60 (ref. pg. 349)
3. 50 (ref. pg. 349)
4. 40 (ref. pg. 350)
5. anaerobic threshold (ref. pg. 350)

VENTILATION

1. a. The cerebral cortex sending neural signals to the exercising muscles may also send collateral signals to the medulla to increase the rate and depth of breathing.
   b. Proprioceptors in the moving muscles, tendons, and joints transmit sensory signals via the spinal cord to the respiratory centers of the medulla.
   c. The increase in body temperature during exercise may also contribute to increased ventilation. (ref. pg. 351)
2. e (ref. pg. 351)
3. depth, rate (ref. pg. 351)
4. depth, frequency (rate) (ref. pg. 351)
5. e (ref. pg. 351)
6. a. an increase in alveolar ventilation, within seconds after the onset of exercise.
   b. a slow, gradual further increase in alveolar ventilation developing over approximately the first 3 minutes of exercise.
   c. alveolar ventilation stabilizes. (ref. pg. 351)

7. 50, 65 (ref. pg. 352)
8. 250 (ref. pg. 352)
9. 95 (ref. pg. 353)
10. c (ref. pg. 353)
11. increased cardiac output (ref. pg. 353)
12. d (ref. pg. 354)

CIRCULATION

1. a. sympathetic discharge
   b. in cardiac output
   c. in arterial blood pressure (ref. pg. 355)
2. a. The heart is stimulated to increase its rate and strength of contraction
   b. The blood vessels of the peripheral vascular system constrict, except for the blood vessels of the working muscles, which dilate (ref. pg. 356)
3. an increased cardiac output (ref. pg. 356)
4. a. an increased stroke volume
   b. an increased heart rate
   c. combination of both (ref. pg. 356)
5. vasodilation (ref. pg. 356)
6. Frank-Starling (ref. pg. 357)
7. 165 (ref. pg. 357)
8. increases, decreases (ref. pg. 351)
9. a. the individual's physical condition
   b. the specific muscles that are working
   c. the distribution of blood flow (ref. pg. 357)
10. decreases (ref. pg. 357)
11. a. the sympathetic discharge
    b. the increased cardiac output
    c. the vasoconstriction of the blood vessels in the non-working muscle areas. (ref. pg. 357)
12. a. increases
    b. increases
    c. increases
    d. increases (ref. pg. 357)
13. local vasodilators (ref. pg. 358)

STROKE VOLUME VERSUS HEART RATE IN INCREASING THE CARDIAC OUTPUT

1. heart rate, increased stroke volume (ref. pg. 360)
2. 50 (ref. pg. 360)
3. increased heart rate (ref. pg. 360)
4. 65 (ref. pg. 360)

BODY TEMPERATURE/CUTANEOUS BLOOD FLOW RELATIONSHIP

1. profuse sweating, followed by no sweating; extreme weakness; muscle cramping; exhaustion; nausea; headache; dizziness; confusion; staggering gait; unconsciousness; circulatory collapse (ref. pg. 361)
2. a. Spraying cool water on the victim's body
   b. Continually sponging the victim with cool water
   c. Blowing air over the body with a strong fan
   d. A combination of all three (ref. pg. 362)

CARDIOVASCULAR REHABILITATION

1. a. acute, inpatient
   b. outpatient, immediately after hospitalization
   c. long-term outpatient
   d. maintenance (ref. pg. 362)

CHAPTER FIFTEEN

HIGH ALTITUDE AND ITS EFFECTS ON THE CARDIOPULMONARY SYSTEM

ANSWERS

EFFECTS OF HIGH ALTITUDE

1. 18,000–19,000 (ref. pg. 367)
2. increased alveolar ventilation (ref. pg. 369)
3. six weeks (ref. pg. 369)
4. c (ref. pg. 369)
5. c (ref. pg. 370)
6. 20–25% greater (ref. pg. 370)
7. a (ref. pg. 370)
8. increased (ref. pg. 370)
9. c (ref. pg. 371)
10. a (ref. pg. 372)

OTHER PHYSIOLOGIC CHANGES

1. a (ref. pg. 373)
2. headache, fatigue, dizziness, palpitation, nausea, loss of appetite, and insomnia (ref. pg. 374)
3. second or third day after ascent (ref. pg. 374)
4. vasoconstriction; increased (ref. pg. 374)
5. photophobia, ataxia, hallucinations, clouding of consciousness, coma, and possibly death (ref. pg. 374)
6. fatigue, reduced exercise tolerance, headache, dizziness, somnolence, loss of mental acuity, marked polycythemia, and severe hypoxemia (ref. pg. 374)

CHAPTER SIXTEEN

HIGH-PRESSURE ENVIRONMENTS AND THEIR EFFECT ON THE CARDIOPULMONARY SYSTEM

ANSWERS

DIVING

1. 1.0 atmosphere (ref. pg. 377)
2. a. 1.375 liters (ref. pg. 378)
   b. 3040 mm Hg (ref. pg. 378)
3. a. the diver's metabolic rate
   b. the diver's ability to store and transport O_2 and CO_2 (ref. pg. 379)
4. 55 (ref. pg. 379)
5. descends, ascends (ref. pg. 379)
6. hypoxia of ascent (ref. pg. 380)
7. a. bradycardia
   b. decreased cardiac output
   c. peripheral vasoconstriction (ref. pg. 380)
8. a. joint pains (the bends)
   b. chest pain and coughing (the chokes)
   c. paresthesia and paralysis (spinal cord involvement)
   d. circulatory failure
   e. death (severe cases) (ref. pg. 380)

HYPERBARIC MEDICINE

1. (ref. pg. 392)
2. a. increases the physically dissolved O_2 in the arterial blood
   b. increases the pressure gradient for driving oxygen into ischemic tissues
   c. reduces the half-life of carboxyhemoglobin (Hb_{CO}) (ref. pg. 383)
3. 1 hour (ref. pg. 383